God bless
You
You Ber

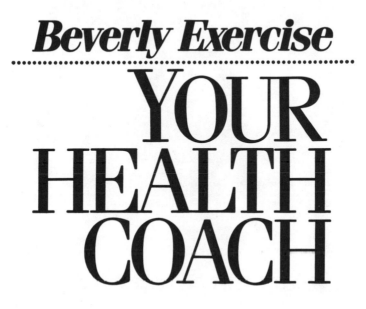

Beverly Exercise

YOUR HEALTH COACH

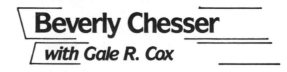

Beverly Chesser
with Gale R. Cox

Beverly Exercise—Your Health Coach

Beverly P. Chesser with Gale R. Cox

Copyright 1988 by Beverly P. Chesser
Printed in the United States of America
ISBN: 0-88368-210-9

*Editorial assistance for Whitaker House by Debra Petrosky.
Cover photo by Darrel Thomas.*

Scripture quotations marked *NIV* are taken from the *New International Version,* copyright © 1973, 1978, 1984, International Bible Society and are used by permission. Scripture quotations marked *KJV* are taken from the *King James Version.*

Dedication

I want to dedicate this book to a number of people who have blessed my life. First, to my husband Ryland Chesser, who married me at probably the lowest point of my life, who refused to let me get fat, and who insisted I join my first exercise class. His love would not allow me to do anything that threatened my well-being.

To Marion McGill, who first boldly witnessed the Lord Jesus Christ to me and gave me that desire to have what she had in her heart.

To Charlie Jones, the on-fire-for-the-Lord pastor who preached the Lord Jesus Christ, led me to repentance, and then taught me God's Holy Word so I could grow and be a witness for the Lord.

To my daughter, Leah Rachel Chesser, who is my heritage from the Lord and who has blessed my life beyond what words can say.

To my mother, who taught all ten of her children to be hardworking and honest. Her submissive spirit to my father exemplified one who has been born again. I never knew how she did it until I became born again and God's Holy Spirit and Word taught me.

To my father, Norman Ashy Payne, who taught me to be a businesswoman and helped me stay in shape—the old-fashioned way.

To my sister, June Breeden, whom I love dearly. June was like a mother to me at times, giving me my first and only birthday party when I desired so much to be accepted by the other children. And for always loving, encouraging, and financially helping me to expand *Beverly Exercise* saying, "You must never give up. God has given you this talent."

To my sister, Marion, who loved me as a child and called me "Pet." When I was a scrawny kid, Marion told me that I was beautiful, smart, and going to turn out "great." She made me believe in myself and made me feel special. She was a registered nurse and died when she was only thirty-three.

To every single one of my viewers who has listened to me, worked with me, put up with my accent, talked back to me, suffered with sore muscles in the beginning, told their friends about me, prayed for me, and financially supported my ministry through donations and tape purchases, *Thank you from the bottom of my heart.*

To all the stations who have aired *Beverly Exercise* as a ministry to their viewers when they could have sold that air time to another ministry: *Thank you and God bless you.*

A very special thank you to WGGS TV-16 in Greenville, South Carolina, who produced my program for two years at no charge as a ministry to their viewers. To Mike Ward of WGGS TV-16 who noticed me on my very first talk show and asked me that very day if I wanted to have my own program. Together with WGGS, Mike put my program on the air.

To WTKK TV-66 who produced and first syndicated *Beverly Exercise* at a time when WGGS TV-16 had to drop production of the show. Both of these stations were the stepping stones God used to get us to a point where we could pay to produce and distribute our program.

Again, to Ryland Chesser, who through all my trials and hard times, stood by me. He believed God had started a good work in me and He would continue it until the day of Jesus Christ, and he wouldn't let me ever think it was time to quit. He has been *my* coach, constantly assuring me that God has anointed and equipped me with serving power and talent.

Acknowledgement

I want to express my deepest appreciation to Robert E. T. Stark, M.D. for his invaluable help and encouragement. His books, *Controlling Fat for Life* and *The Percent Fat Calories Tables* provided the incentive I needed to finish this manuscript. His books and subsequent words of encouragement renewed my resolve and commitment to spread the word about good health and life-long weight control through low-fat eating and regular exercise.

Thank you, Dr. Stark.

Foreword

The American "health care system" is in a continuing state of crisis with respect to ever increasing costs and diminishing returns. As the nation spends more money on the system, there is no evident increase in the health of its citizens. There is no marked decrease in the prevalency of heart disease, stroke, hypertension, diabetes mellitus, cancers, and other chronic diseases.

A significant part of the health care problem is that we really do not have a health care system as such. In the United States we have excellent providers of medical, surgical, and hospital care; however, they do not provide *health* care.

The concept of a health care system implies that somewhere in the system we can find health if we look hard enough. If we continue to rely on the system for our health, our society will continue to be disappointed, frustrated, and critical of the results.

The two principal deficits in our so-called health care system are the lack of emphasis on disease and injury prevention and the almost absent emphasis on individual responsibility for health. These two factors are frequently intertwined. Lung cancer due to cigarette smoking and automobile injuries due to excessive speed, not wearing seat belts or drunken driving are just two examples.

Obesity, the number one preventable medical problem in America, affects over 20 percent of our adult population. In the vast majority of cases, obesity is a preventable medical disease. Carrying excess weight is associated with many serious, chronic medical disorders such as coronary artery disease, adult onset diabetes, and many types of cancer.

The costs to society for treatment of obesity and its associated illnesses are mind boggling. Dr. George Blackburn of Harvard University Medical School has estimated that the elimination of obesity would reduce the total costs of all medical, surgical, and hospital costs by 25 percent!

The probability of finding medical and financial relief from the staggering costs of treating preventable medical problems such as obesity in our health care system is at the present time remote. One reason is the failure of our government, the medical insurance agency, and organized medicine to recognize obesity as a specific disease entity.

If we can't find effective solutions for obesity in the health care system, we must seek help elsewhere. If we, as a nation, are ever going to get a handle on the increasing financial burdens of the current system, we must look to ourselves, which means taking more individual responsibility for our health and for the individual behaviors that effect it. We can no longer afford to rely on a health care system that was never designed to provide or deliver health.

I believe most Americans desire to take better command of their health. Witness the remarkable upsurge in fitness centers and the proliferation of diet and self-help books. The fact that large corporations are establishing exercise centers for their employees, that many of us are working out in aerobics and dance centers, and that we are reading and making bestsellers of books on food strategies and weight control, acknowledges our deeply felt need for sound advice, counseling, and guidance.

The key to intelligent decisions about essential requisites for good health is information, especially up-to-date information on sensible nutrition and physical fitness. If we are going to enjoy good health, we need to eat and exercise sensibly. These are the two principal requirements for weight control and good health.

We now have documented information about what constitutes sound nutrition, which is quite different from the conventional wisdom of the past thirty years. We are also learning more about the value of exercise and its relationship to maintenance of good health and disease avoidance.

Before aerobics and fitness programs became fashionable, Beverly pioneered exercise programs for television audiences and began a study of nutrition principles. Through her television program, *Beverly Exercise,* and her audio and video tapes on exercise and physical fitness, she has built up a national audience. Beverly utilizes her unique status as a television celebrity to coach her television audience on the merits of good health and how to achieve it.

After twenty years of coaching thousands on health matters, she has written her first book, *Beverly Exercise— Your Health Coach,* in which she shares her personal life experiences and the knowledge that she has gained as a wife, mother, teacher, and counselor. Her book is a valuable contribution to the literature on fitness and health.

I know you will benefit from the wisdom and maturity that Beverly has earned through her years of hard work and dedication to mental, physical, and spiritual health.

Robert E. T. Stark, M.D.

Dr. Stark is a past president of The American Society of Bariatric Physicians (doctors who treat obese patients and their associated medical problems). He is also the author of several books and has had articles published in medical journals and national magazines.

Contents

Part One
Beverly's Story

How difficult it is to get through the day when we are burdened with unhealthy bodies! I know because I've been there.

This book is meant to be a reference source on good nutrition and health—based on my own experiences and study. My prayer is that this book will help you have a healthy life that truly glorifies our Lord Jesus Christ.

1

Ups and Downs

I was born into a family that included my father, mother, a grandmother, and ten brothers and sisters. Growing up, I knew little else but work—hard work.

At age eleven, I began accompanying my father on Saturdays with his egg route in Alexandria, Virginia. We loaded the truck with cases of eggs and drove sixty miles from Culpeper to Alexandria. Carrying two buckets loaded down with eggs, I sold them door-to-door to our egg customers who called me "the little egg girl."

My personality began to develop as I learned how to talk to people and maintain good working relationships. Some customers let me walk right into their houses and put the eggs in their refrigerators. At Christmas time I received so many gifts from appreciative customers that I shared my presents with my little brother and sisters.

Being an "egg girl" was excellent business training. I sold nearly two hundred dollars' worth of eggs every Saturday, making me a major contributor to the family income. Handling money and keeping a book of credit when the customers were unable to pay were excellent skills to learn.

Because there was no one to take my place, I couldn't even be sick. From that time through my eleventh year of high school, I was faithful to my egg route, never once missing a Saturday. This created a problem with the band leader, however, since I was a clarinetist in the marching and concert bands. When our high school band was scheduled to perform on Saturdays, I could never go along. The egg business came first.

Recalling this time in my life, I remember how my peers made fun of me and called me names. The memories of my adolescent years are painful ones. I loved the adults, but the children were unkind to me.

Daddy used to tease me and say that I was going to make some man a wonderful wife—tending the chickens and raising babies. I told him, "I will never be a farmer's wife. I'm getting off this farm as soon as I can!" The problem was I didn't know how—not until the day Daddy brought home our first black and white television.

Della Street and Me

When I saw the *Perry Mason* program, a young lady named Della Street caught my eye. She was so efficient, and everyone depended on her. Della kept everything organized and always had the right answers. That was what I wanted to be—a Della Street in somebody's office.

That summer I talked Daddy into buying me a typewriter and a typing book, and I taught myself to type. I knew I had finally discovered the way to get off the farm.

The fall following my summer crash course in typing, I was determined to do everything possible to graduate from high school with enough knowledge to get a job in Washington, D.C. The first nine weeks were pretty standard for me in typing. We learned the basic keyboard, and I moved along at the same pace as everyone else. The teacher never suspected that I had mastered the keyboard and had even taught myself to type sixty correct words per minute.

The fun began the second nine weeks. I'll never forget it! We had a bulletin board project assigned to us. On this bulletin board, up in the right hand corner, was the moon. Down at the bottom of the left hand corner were individual rocket ships bearing the name of each member of the class. At specific points on the board were goals representing typing speed—twenty, thirty, forty, fifty, and sixty correct words per minute. The object was to reach the moon and type sixty correct words per minute.

The teacher gave our first test. "On your mark, get set, go!" Everyone began typing furiously. Many students stumbled with their fingers on the wrong keys, others lost time looking at their papers, and some just panicked. Not me. I had practiced with that time clock all summer. I kept my cool, and when the teacher yelled "Stop!" I had completed her assignment.

I have never seen a teacher so surprised. Many of the other students had received an "A" the first nine weeks, and I had received only a "B." Because we weren't tested, the teacher had only assumed who her "A" students were. That day my teacher assured me that I was a champion, and she never let me forget it.

She encouraged me to schedule commercial courses so I would be able to get a good job after graduation. At her insistence I joined the Future Business Leaders of America, and even competed for Miss FBLA. Winning the local contest in Culpeper and then the Regional Miss FBLA Contest at Madison College in Harrisonburg, Virginia, was a thrill.

In each of these contests I was interviewed first by businessmen and then by college professors. Many wondered how a farm girl like me could do so well. They didn't know that I had several years of business experience behind me.

Where Do I Go from Here?

After graduation from high school, I landed a job in Washington, D.C. and married my childhood sweetheart.

But the nine years that followed were some of the most painful years of my life. We struggled through career changes, several moves, military service for my husband, and financial stress, but I always managed to keep the problems to myself.

Then my husband left me, and suddenly I had to face the burden of paying financial debts, selling a house, and establishing myself as a single woman. Coming from a home where divorce was totally unacceptable, my personal situation became more than I could handle.

I lived on black coffee and cigarettes. With finances so tight, food didn't interest me, and I tended to view this as a blessing. People kept telling me I had lost a lot of weight. I loved the attention, so I didn't bother to eat. Besides, I could never seem to set aside money for groceries. Once, after going for three days without food, it suddenly occurred to me, "Hey, you haven't eaten lately!"

I also remember thinking, "This is great. I don't have to eat!" Actually, I was borderline anorexic and didn't even realize it. The brain of an anorexic will tell her that she does not need to eat.

Bald and Toothless?

I probably would have totally wasted away had not two things happened. My hair started falling out, and my teeth became loose. My doctor insisted that I start eating again because my body fat content was dangerously low. "Beverly, you must take care of yourself. Exercise, eat right, and quit smoking!" I knew he was right. Something had to be done because I had reached an all-time low of 79 pounds!

No longer secretly pleased with my tiny figure, I began picturing myself bald and toothless. Terrified by those thoughts, I got down on my knees and prayed. At that time in my life, I only prayed if I couldn't handle something alone. Up to this point, I had mostly thought of God as somebody "up there" just waiting to nail me. Little did I know that because of my pitiful circumstances, God would someday use me to help others with the same problems.

My hair and teeth were just the beginning of my health problems. My sinuses were blocked all the time, and a constant drainage irritated the back of my throat. Every morning began with clearing my throat and feeling nauseated. I also broke out in hives from my face all the way down to my feet.

When I sought medical help, I learned I was allergic to ninety different substances. That was the beginning of an allergy shot program that lasted ten years. In addition, I had to use inhalents and take allergy medications. Allergies are dangerous and can even be life-threatening. Twice I had to be rushed to the emergency room of the hospital for adrenalin. The doctor said if my pressure points had been different, I would have died before receiving treatment.

"Beverly," he said, "you have a dangerous condition. You better stay close to the Lord because if you are ever hit at the right pressure point, you will be a goner."

Dangerous Dieting

During this time I married my present husband, Ryland Chesser. Ryland began to see that I ate well, and I started to regain some needed weight. Not knowing much about exercise, I expected to add pounds in all the right places. Before starving myself, I had a near-perfect shape even though I didn't exercise. Heredity and nature had not caught up with me yet. While the scales indicated healthy weight gain, my mirror revealed a serious problem. A size one, junior petite fit me across the shoulders, but I needed size nine/ten slacks to accommodate my spreading hips and thighs! I had lost lean muscle mass and fluid, but the regained weight was quickly deposited in my fat cells.

I began to force my body to lose weight. Working full time made it easy to skip breakfast and lunch. After coming home absolutely starved, I gorged myself on dinner. If I caved in to hunger after fasting for several days, my appetite careened out of control. During my binges I ate everything in the house! After the massive feeding session was over, I mentally beat myself, promising to totally abstain from food. This is called "yo-yo" dieting.

Finding a doctor who believed in diuretics only made matters worse. When my weight was up, taking a water pill allowed me to effortlessly shed five pounds! I was also unknowingly depleting my body of potassium. Despite feeling so weak that I could hardly walk after taking a water pill, I decided wobbly legs were better than being fat.

Maintaining my weight around 100 pounds may have been a source of pride, but my shape certainly wasn't like it used to be. Forcing myself into jeans was a depressing, unsuccessful ordeal. If I found a pair that could slide past my spreading thighs, they were too big in the waist and seat. I remember standing in front of the mirror and crying because I couldn't control my body. What was I going to do?

My Turning Point

During this time, Ryland was watching what was going on in my life. He knew I was desperately hooked on cigarettes, which were only worsening my allergies. One day he called me aside and told me what I did not want to hear. "Beverly, your sisters are heavy and they are happy enough with the way they look, but you are different. You will never be happy as long as you're in poor shape." He told me to join a fitness center and begin exercising.

How I hated those words! I thought he had married me for better or for worse. Now, because I was getting fat, he was trying to change me. First I cried, then I went to the spa.

If you have ever been to a spa, you'll know exactly what I'm about to describe. A sleek, shapely woman wearing a french-cut leotard greets you at the door. She measures you in places where you have never been measured before. Then she bounces you on a scale and writes your weight and personal dimensions in large print on a personal profile chart. Next, she plans your activity sheet for you. By then, you want to crawl under the rug! As you start your exercises, you feel as if life has somehow betrayed you.

I felt so foolish, and I despised exercising. On the farm we were taught to work every minute and to keep our home in order. When you've been raised to exercise only through hard work, you feel guilty when you take time off just to do sit-ups in a room full of women in leotards. After being at work all day, I felt I needed to be home with my husband and doing my household chores in the evening.

Yet I knew I had to come to terms with my physical condition. Without regular exercise and weight control, I was not going to be good for anyone. My husband could not stand to see me starving and then beating myself mentally every time I had anything to eat. I knew I had to give this exercise program my whole heart, not just part of it.

Head of the Class

At the spa, I went right through my program using all the equipment, but I wasn't sure about the "floor exercises." They looked so foolish to me.

One particular exercise really looked strange. We were down on our knees with our arms straight and palms flat to the floor. We were told to bring one knee in close to our head and then kick the other leg out and up—sort of like a mule. That was the name of the exercise—"mule kick."

I really didn't want to do that one because it reminded me of the farm I had so desperately wanted to leave. But my teacher told me the floor work would really shape my hips and thighs, and that was where I needed the most work. Reminding myself that my total heart had to be in the program, I began to kick like a mule.

I was extremely sore after two days of exercise! By the end of the week my muscles still ached, but I was convinced that this was my body's way of telling me I needed work. At the end of the two weeks, I could feel a difference! Stamina and strength had begun to replace that tired feeling that continually dragged me down.

Soon I had worked my way to the head of the exercise class. Standing in front of the teacher, I wanted to exercise right in order to receive the maximum benefit. I was becoming a real believer in exercise and soon had to have my daily exercise "fix."

I began getting up early and exercising. I started walking, riding my bike, and exercising with a lady on TV who wasn't very nice. But I exercised with her anyway because the "new" Beverly was feeling good.

Size Three, Junior Petite

I will never forget that first scheduled time for remeasuring and weighing at the spa. I had been working out faithfully for two months. My entire body had shed inches and pounds, but the most noticeable improvement was in my hips and thighs where I lost four inches!

Even before they measured me, my weight loss was obvious because I could easily slip into my size three, junior petite jeans. It was wonderful! Because I have exercised faithfully since the day I began—now close to twenty years ago—I wear those same jeans today.

The more fit I became, the more I became convicted of what cigarettes were doing to me. I had cut back on smoking but desired to get them totally out of my life. Once that commitment was made, I exercised, drank water, or took a deep breath to combat my craving for nicotine. I also avoided coffee and highly-seasoned foods that brought on a desire for cigarettes. Cutting out cigarettes was difficult at first, but exercise was the perfect replacement for this bad habit. My desire for cigarettes gradually decreased.

Six months after beginning my fitness program, I was like a new person! I felt as if the weight of the world had lifted off my shoulders. I wanted to proclaim "fitness" to the world! I wanted everyone I met to know that they could be free. Why, just six months before, I had been taking two allergy shots a week and had all the indications of asthma. Now, even the doctors were amazed at the new me.

A New Addition

At age thirty-two, I unexpectantly became pregnant. Having been told that I would never have children, I was thrilled at the news. Rapid weight gain at the onset of my pregnancy, however, caused me to suspect a diabetic condition. I gained seven pounds in six weeks! A glucose tolerance test confirmed my suspicion—I had diabetes.

My pregnancy had to be a very controlled one. I had to watch everything I ate. With proper diet and exercise, however, I delivered my baby girl naturally. As I look back over my pregnancy now, I can see the big part daily exercise (floor exercises and walking) played in keeping me physically sound during my pregnancy. A strong body tolerates pregnancy better.

Every female should avoid abnormal weight gain during puberty and pregnancy. The fat cells laid down during these periods of rapid growth will never go away. They may shrink with proper exercise and diet, but they never go away entirely.

After Leah's birth I began a stressful struggle to be a perfect mother—something none of us can come close to being without God's help. While trying so very hard to be good, I was tormented with questions about God, life, and my past.

I carried a deep fear that somehow God might punish me for my past, and I was afraid He would use Leah to get to me. What a wrong picture I had of God! How much I had to learn about His mercy, love, and forgiveness!

2

The New Beverly

When Leah was born, I really wanted to "do right." I had done a lot of bad things in my life, but with the added responsibilities of being a parent, I wanted to make a change.

All my life I had played with religion. Since childhood I had attended Sunday School and church, but as I grew older my attendance slackened. I often experienced pangs of guilt for not going because I had been brought up to be in church every Sunday.

When I went to church, I felt the weight of conviction for my sin. Despite my vow to turn over a new leaf, I found myself repeatedly falling into the same sins and habits. I couldn't seem to gain control of my life.

One Sunday morning, out of appreciation for the day care program they provided for my daughter, I attended the services of a local church. Leah was doing well in their day care, and her caregiver was always glad to see us every morning when we arrived.

The woman who kept Leah was nice, but I just knew something had to be wrong with her because she was continually saying, "Praise the Lord!" She couldn't seem to speak more than five sentences without praising the Lord for something. I knew it took a real nut to do that, but she sure was a great baby tender.

The joy of the Lord in her heart also showed on her face. As this woman demonstrated Christ's love to my daughter and me, I realized that I lacked the spiritual power in my life that she possessed. She made me want what she had!

Where Was I Going?

I had no idea what to expect during my first visit to that new church. The young, Texan pastor warned the congregation of hell and damnation! He preached about the blood of Jesus. At the end of the service, he even asked everyone who knew they were going to heaven to raise their hands. Everyone's hand shot up except Ryland's and mine.

I was afraid the next question would be, "How many know they are going down below?" and I would be forced to raise my hand. I knew my sins outweighed my good deeds, disqualifying me for heaven.

I left church that Sunday really troubled. They certainly didn't make me feel that bad in the church I had previously been attending, so I decided not to return to that Baptist church.

Well, guess who came calling that week? Yes, good old Pastor Jones. Boy, did he ask some embarrassing questions! He even had the audacity to say I could *know* if I was going to heaven.

Having been troubled all my life with dying, cemetaries, and hell, I really listened. Pastor Jones shared the gospel of Jesus Christ with me for over three hours. For every question and objection I raised, he had an answer—Jesus Christ. Pastor Jones believed I was saved but lacked the blessed assurance that I was going to heaven.

We finally got rid of Pastor Jones that night by promising him we would visit his church again the following Sunday. All week I felt crushed beneath the weight of my guilt and hemmed in by the pressure of conviction. In anguish I wrestled with my spiritual condition. More than anything I wanted that blessed assurance of being saved.

What an impassioned message Pastor Jones preached the following Sunday! That morning, I felt compelled to go forward and ask Jesus into my heart. God had tarried with me long enough. Knowing what Jesus had done for me through Calvary, I couldn't wait another moment to be saved. I walked the aisle, knelt at the altar, and asked Jesus Christ to be my Lord and Savior.

Gifts from God

From that moment on I've experienced a hunger for God's Word and a desire to bring others to Jesus. I knew there were folks out there just like me—lost as could be—just taking up space in churches. I wanted them to know the saving and sanctifying power of Jesus.

Before I was saved, the most eloquent, animated preacher couldn't move me. But after I was saved, the Bible became a new book to me. Suddenly the pages of Scripture were filled with excitement and priceless nuggets of truth.

My first Bible study on 1 Peter taught me to reverence and submit to my husband. Ryland told Pastor Jones that reverencing and submitting would be a new experience for me. I admitted to myself, "Maybe this is the reason I'm already in a second marriage."

My previous problems had surfaced because I had not followed God's plan for marriage. Through studying the Scriptures, I discovered new truths and found power for my life. Seeing my husband and daughter as gifts from God helped me to love and appreciate them even more.

Drowning My Sorrows

Shortly after I was saved, we decided to move to Anderson, South Carolina, due to my husband's continued heart problems. I weighed 98 pounds and was in good spiritual and physical shape. It never occurred to me that there were still more battles to be fought.

We moved into a house that needed lots of repairs; my husband was ill; and I had a small child to care for. In no time at all the smallest irritations began to upset me. When I got upset, guess what I would do? Right. I would eat. I also missed the exercise teacher I had in New Jersey. How did I cope with my frustrations? Where did I find my comfort? I began to drown my sorrows in food—lots of food.

Ryland soon became wise to me. One day when he was walking out the door, he remarked, "I'm going to the mall, and I want you to try not to eat everything in the house while I'm gone." I thought I would die!

As soon as he left, I headed straight for the refrigerator and just packed the food away. At the very moment I finished eating, I said to myself, "I'd better read the Bible. I haven't had my quiet time today." I had been committed to my eating time but not my quiet time. Better let the Lord in on this, right? Ease the guilt a little.

I opened up the Bible and immediately my eyes fell on the Scripture, "Put a knife to your throat if you are given to gluttony" (Proverbs 23:2, NIV). I gasped and thought, "Oh, Lord! You really do watch all the time!"

When Jesus Christ comes into your heart, He goes everywhere you go. If I'm into gluttony in the kitchen, He's there with me. If I'm exercising, He's there, too.

Kneeling on my face before God, right then and there, I repented. "Heavenly Father, I am such a sinner. I know how to exercise, and I know how to walk tall for You. Please forgive me for not glorifying You in my eating. From this day on, help me to eat as You would have me to."

Giving Myself a Gift

God had blessed me with a husband and a beautiful daughter, and I had let my health go. The day of my repentance,

I tipped the scales at 114 pounds and wore size ten pants. That may not seem like much to most people, but for someone who is small-boned and only five feet, two inches tall, it was traumatic. In less than four months my weight had ballooned from 98 to 114 pounds. I felt as though the life was being crushed out of me between walls of fat.

Beginning that day, I promised to exercise every day for God's glory. Forgetting the tape measure and the scales, I just purposed in my heart to glorify God in my body. My emotions would no longer control me. In my weak areas, I began to let the power of God guide me. It was not easy. It was work. And I worked!

Finally ready to do things God's way, the idea of giving myself the gifts of fitness and health gradually became a reality. In addition to joining an exercise class, I began jogging and biking as well. My lifestyle changed as I read books on nutrition and began to plan balanced meals.

Exercise as a Ministry?

At the health club I joined in Anderson, a preacher's wife saw me exercising. When she saw how trained I was, she began urging me to offer exercise classes for the women of her church. I tried to ignore her suggestions, but she pressed the issue until I agreed.

With some reluctance and uncertainty I began classes at the church, secretly telling myself, "If I work them hard enough, they won't come back." But they all returned and brought friends with them.

Up until that time, God had not revealed any special gift or calling on my life. But two weeks into the program I felt that God had placed me in a ministry. I asked my pastor, "Could this be possible? Whoever heard of an exercise ministry?"

He replied, "Beverly, I believe all those years when you were out there playing Della Street and going to exercise classes in the evening, the Lord was preparing you for this ministry."

In no time at all, I was presenting exercise programs at five churches. Word spread. Soon I was called to be on a local TV program to share my testimony and demonstrate my work.

While on this program, I mentioned that I made cassette tapes of exercise classes for those who were unable to attend a class in person. So many calls for those tapes came in during the program that afterward the producer came to me and said, "I'm going to talk to the owners and see if we can't start an exercise show. Would you be interested in doing it?"

"Oh, no," I immediately responded, "I'm going to be thirty-nine on my next birthday."

But at the same moment I was also aware of God's providential hand in the matter. So I said, "Wait a minute. Yes, I will do a pilot show and leave the rest up to the Lord."

I went home and prayed, "Lord, if You want me to have an exercise program, give me the Holy Spirit power to really pour out my testimony."

And it happened! I began taping my exercise show. My husband would get copies of each show we made at WGGS TV-16 in Greenville, South Carolina, and he would take these to other stations. Soon new stations were adding my program to their line-up.

Beverly Exercise

Now my show is seen nationwide on several satellite networks and hundreds of independent stations. The program is produced through Beverly Exercise TV Corporation, a non-profit Christian corporation.

And what is so thrilling is the "miracle" of it all! If I had ever planned to do this on my own, I would have surely failed. For one thing, I could never have financed such a project. Only God could have brought it about. All I had to do was be willing to be used of the Lord.

During the show I help viewers exercise, encourage them to develop healthy lifestyles, and share the love of Jesus. I speak from experience. I've been where so many of them are (and where *you* may be now)—sick, depressed, and looking to food for answers. I know what it's like to battle your body without discipline and to face life without Jesus.

Satan tried to kill me and render me useless to God, but Christ came in and gave me victory and abundant life. Praise God! "The thief cometh not, but for to steal, and to kill, and to destroy: I am come that they might have life, and that they might have it more abundantly" (John 10:10, KJV).

Your Health Coach *Reread*

Looking back, I can see where I had to get physically strong before I realized how spiritually weak and totally empty I was. God placed me in the ministry of exercise in order to teach people that a healthy spirit, body, and mind go together. Each is needed in order for the others to function properly. A healthy body will not stay healthy long if the spirit or mind is sick.

Through Christ, I gained victory over poor health, lack of self-esteem, and guilt. And so can you. God wants us to glorify Him in all we say and do. He wants discipline in our lives. We must glorify Him in the care and exercise of our bodies and in the way we eat. This only comes about as we truly see ourselves as God's special creations.

I believe the Lord has given every person a fantastic amount of potential—all we have to do is use it. Looking in the mirror at bulging thighs and hips can discourage anybody. Cultivate a positive attitude. Begin now to thank the Lord for your wonderful body. Tell Him, "I know that with Your help, Lord, I can lose weight and be healthy."

I pray God will use this book to help you become a total, whole people for Jesus. In the chapters that follow, let me be your health coach and together we can glorify God.

——Part Two——
Smart Dieting

—3—
The Fat You Eat is the Fat You Wear

One purpose of this book is to train you to spot the fat in your diet and reduce the amount you are consuming.

Remember, the fat you see on your plate is the fat you will see on your body. If you eat it, you will wear it. Once you learn to spot fat in your food, you can eliminate it and eventually enjoy a slimmer, healthier body—without being hungry all the time. Begin to ask yourself daily, "Where are the fats hiding in my diet?"

By the time you finish reading this book, I believe you will be so informed that your mind will act like a calculator when you look at food. You will know exactly what foods you can eat to keep from gaining weight and what foods you must avoid.

Facts on Fat

The foods we eat are divided into three categories—fats, carbohydrates, and proteins. If you want to be healthy and maintain an ideal weight, how should you balance your foods?

—55 percent of your total calories should be complex carbohydrates (fruits, whole grains, and vegetables);
—not over 30 percent of calories should be fat;
—the balance of your calories should be protein.

Why cut back on fat? Fats are the most concentrated source of energy in your diet, containing twice the calories found in carbohydrates and proteins. Each gram of fat contains *nine* calories, compared to *four* calories per gram for carbohydrates and protein. *Forty percent* of the average American's daily calorie intake is fat.

Fat has three main functions: to carry Vitamins A, D, E, and K; to provide cushion and protection for the body's vital organs; and to insulate the body. Fat also improves the taste of food. We do need fat in our diets—but in regulated amounts.

If you control your fat intake and exercise regularly, you will be able to maintain a correct weight once that set weight has been reached. Identifying the fat in your diet, substituting better food in its place, and exercising will do wonders for your health.

How Fat Makes You Fat

Foods high in fat stay in the stomach longer than low-fat foods. The stomach usually empties within three hours following a meal, but fried potatoes may still be in your stomach the next day.

Complex carbohydrates, such as vegetables, fruits, whole grains, greens, and pasta will digest easily and quickly, but high-fat foods require more stomach digestion. If you eat when you are worried, afraid, or nervous, the food will stay in your stomach longer. Each person requires a different amount of time for digestion.

Fat makes you fat because it slows the digestion and absorption of food. In experiments where animals were fed a totally fat diet, they had zero metabolism (or conversion of food to energy) after eating. The activity of the body was so low it was as if they had not eaten at all.

Most of the fat we eat on our plates is stored as fat on our bodies. The average American consumes as much as eight times more fat per day than what is actually needed. Our bodies need the fat equivalent of only one tablespoon of vegetable oil each day. On the other hand, too little fat can lead to a deficiency in the fat-soluble vitamins A,D,E, and K, which may lead to various ailments that will be discussed in the chapter on vitamins.

Too much fat, of course, causes weight gain and a slowing of the digestion and proper absorption of food. Excess fat leads to the storage of abnormal amounts of cholesterol throughout the body, which contributes to heart disease, high blood pressure, stroke, and various others serious illnesses.

Fat Cells

Fats are broken into two categories: *essential fats* and *stored fats*. Essential fats are present in the brain, spinal cord, and various other internal organs. Storage fats are located mainly below the skin and are used for insulation and protection of vital organs. Storage fat is the largest source of fuel for your body. When the number of calories you eat exceeds the number of calories you use, the excess is stored as fat.

Storage fat is in fat cells and generally fills the cells to about half capacity. When the amount of storage fat increases, so does the size of the fat cells in which it is stored. The *number* of the fat cells, however, does not increase. The quantity of fat cells is established early in life and rarely changes.

Obese people have greater amounts of fat per fat cell and three times the average number of fat cells. With weight loss, the size of each fat cell is reduced, but the number of fat cells appears to remain the same. This explains why it is so easy to regain lost weight—the same old fat cells are still there ready to collect.

Brown and White Fat

The body has two kinds of fat—one is stored, the other is used for fuel. Stored fat is often called "white" fat and fuel fat is often called "brown" fat.

Eating triggers the body to release insulin, which stimulates the action of brown fat. Brown fat stimulates body heat and the burning of calories. Our levels of brown fat seem to be genetically determined. This may account for the fact that two people can eat the same food and one will gain weight on it and the other won't. Cold temperatures also activate brown fat, causing it to radiate heat and burn calories.

When you cut back on your eating through dieting, the action of brown fat will decrease and the body temperature will be lowered by the brain in an effort to conserve fuel. Brown fat is a protective mechanism of the body to maintain a steady weight.

You can make your brown fat work for you in weight control. By eating more complex carbohydrates and less fat, and by exercising regularly, you can increase the calorie-burning action of brown fat. This allows your body's caloric thermostat to let off steam.

How Fat Accumulates

Fat may prefer certain locations in your body to other areas. You may be carrying entirely too much storage fat on your buttocks, for example, while being much leaner on the rest of your body. Many dieters also report greater ease in losing from some areas than others.

Fat build-up seems to be dictated by the ratio between two types of receptors found on the surface of fat cells.

Beta-1 receptors stimulate fat breakdown; *alpha-2 receptors* inhibit loss of fat.

A special type of fat cell tends to hoard fat and does not release it easily. Some cells store fat readily and give it up easily. *Fat miser cells,* however, hang on to their fat. When you diet, body fat is released from regular fat cells first and from the fat miser cells last.

Men tend to have fat miser cells over the abdomen, making them more prone to a large expanding middle. Women have fat miser cells over the buttocks and upper thighs. The fat-holding alpha receptors explain why women gain in hips and thighs and men gain in the stomach.

Scientists are beginning to understand the body's fat storage codes and why we gain where we do. Some day knowledge may become available that will enable a person to slim down only in those areas where they have the most fat.

But until more research is done, there is little a person can do to alter his fat-cell receptors except exercise and control fat intake. Exercise does help shift the receptor ratio towards fat breakdown.

What About Cellulite?

The bulged, bumpy fat that collects just under the skin on the hips, thighs, and buttocks is known as cellulite. Cellulite is nothing more than rippled fat. It's not some special kind of fat that has to be dealt with in some special way.

The bumpy, waffle-like appearance of cellulite is caused by the connective tissue that envelops each fat cell and separates those cells into compartments. Since these compartments are just below the skin, your stored fat is quite obvious.

Women are most afflicted with the obvious bumps and humps of cellulite because their outer layer of skin is thinner and their fat compartments larger and more rounded than those of men. Women also tend to deposit fat on their hip and thigh areas where it is more obvious than in the waist area where men deposit theirs.

Older people also appear to have cellulite because of thinning and losing flexibility in the outer layer of skin. Some experts think there may be a genetic tendency toward cellulite, but it does not usually appear unless there is an excess amount of fat in the diet. Like ordinary fat, cellulite can be burned and lost through exercise and low-fat dieting.

Many people who have areas of cellulite think they can get rid of it through "spot reduction." But focusing on just your problem areas is not the way to lose cellulite. You will experience more success in your battle with cellulite by devoting yourself to a well-rounded program of daily exercise. Walking, swimming, and jogging burn more calories per minute than exercises designed for spot reduction.

How Much Fat Is Too Much?

The fat content in the body of a healthy, young woman of normal weight should measure 22 to 26 percent of her total body weight. For example, a 124-pound woman is probably carrying 31 pounds (25 percent) of fat, comprised of four pounds of essential fat and 27 pounds of stored fat. An unacceptable ratio is when storage fat exceeds 30 percent of the body's weight. With this extra fat come flabby arms and jiggly thighs.

If you are near-normal weight, your body contains 25 to 35 billion fat cells—cells that began to develop three months prior to birth and continue to form through adolescence. When the fat content begins to exceed 30 percent of the total body weight, the excess fat begins to engorge those already-existing fat cells. When they reach their limit of endurance, more fat cells develop to handle the overload. This is how an obese person can develop as many as 300 billion fat cells by adulthood.

You may be wondering if you carry too high a percentage of fat cells and how you can measure this. Although there are several ways to supposedly measure the concentration of fat in your body, just look in the mirror. If you see jiggles and flab you have a problem. Save yourself a lot of time and money. Just stand naked in front of the mirror and decide for yourself if you are too fat.

What Causes A Protruding Tummy?

Did you know there is as much fat inside the stomach as under the skin? Regardless of how strong your abdominal muscles are, there is no way to compress internal fat. The following example will demonstrate this point. Fill a plastic bag full of butter and then try to compress the bag. It won't work. A protruding tummy is caused by fat accumulation, and you can't get rid of it without getting rid of internal fat.

How can this be done?

> 1. *Eliminate the excess fat in your diet.* Crazy diets don't work and usually cause you to get fatter when the dieting stops. Just follow a sensible, low-fat diet.
> 2. *Exercise* is absolutely essential to successful fat loss. Exercise burns fat from all over your body. Muscle building exercises help preserve muscle and keep your metabolism going strong. Letting your muscles atrophy will cause your body to burn fewer calories, resulting in excess poundage.

Although most of the time a protruding tummy is caused by poor muscle tone combined with fat, other factors can contribute. Fluid accumulation is a common cause, especially in women who experience premenstrual tension. Congestive heart failure and liver disease also cause accumulation of fluid in the abdomen.

One significant but often overlooked cause for a protruding tummy is the shrinking spine. As the spine shrinks through osteoporosis, the abdominal cavity can maintain its size and hold all the organs only by letting the abdomen protrude. When the spine is bowed, the stomach protrudes. When exercising, keep your back straight and your shoulders back to maintain good posture. Body alignment exercises can prevent the shoulders from rounding and slumping forward.

Where Is Fat Hiding?

Fats are found in meats. These are known as saturated fats. Dairy products are also heavy-fat sources. Cheese is high in fat. Begin to read labels. You'll notice that coconut and palm oil, two saturated fats that should be avoided, are listed in many prepared foods.

Always buy low-fat milk products. Foods like butter, margarine, and mayonnaise are fats. Most grocery stores carry regular mayonnaise and "light" mayonnaise. Look at the mayonnaise selections and pick the one lowest in fat.

One fat that slips by us all the time is salad dressing. Loading up on regular dressing at a salad bar will not save you calories at all. Bacon bits, cheese, and various salads mixed with mayonnaise are high in fat. Carefully select your salad ingredients and then top it with a low-calorie dressing.

Fats are inevitably found in sweets. Cakes, pastries, and cookies contain sugar, and sugar's best friend is fat. Wherever you find sugar, you will find butter and other fat-rich ingredients. Substituting fresh fruits for rich, sweet desserts will remove a big hunk of the fat from your diet.

The Truth About Milk

Milk is very important to your health, but did you know that even low-fat milk is high in fat? Skim milk, which is low in fat and provides all the calcium of whole milk, is really your best choice. I drink skim milk three times a day.

—in whole milk, 54 percent of the calories come from fat;
—in 2 percent milk, 38 percent of the calories come from fat;
—in 1 percent milk, 18 percent of the calories come from fat;
—in 2 percent chocolate milk, 21 percent of the calories come from fat. Skim milk contains only a trace of fat, and is obviously the best choice for adults. Buttermilk also has only a trace of fat.

Were you surprised to learn that 2 percent milk contains so much fat? You may be asking, "How can this be? The label says only 2 percent fat!" What you see on the label and what the milk actually supplies are two different things. Two-percent milk does contain 2 percent butterfat by weight, but milk is mostly water. Since the water in milk provides little nutritional value, defining the fat content in relation to the water content or weight is misleading.

If you want to know how much fat is really in 2 percent milk, read the fine print on the label. Two percent milk supplies 120 calories and 5 grams of fat per cup. Since a gram of fat supplies 9 calories, you can multiply the 5 grams of fat in the milk by 9 and get 45 calories of fat. That means that 45 of the 120 calories in 2 percent milk come from fat. To put it another way, 2 percent milk is 38 percent fat. *Any food over 30 percent fat is considered high-fat.*

Begin to read labels. Pay close attention to the number of fat grams contained in any food. By spotting the fat, you can begin to reduce it in your diet. Remember that *the fat you eat is the fat you will wear.*

4

Outsmarting Your Fat Cells

If you are an adult, you can totally *eliminate* some fats from your diet and neither you nor your body will miss them. Why? Because we eat so much more fat than we need.

We cannot eliminate all fats from our diet, but those we do eliminate must be replaced with something better. Otherwise, we will starve. By replacing fats with complex carbohydrates, we can gain greater control over our weight and health.

Calories from complex carbohydrates and protein actually speed up your metabolism or the way your body uses food for energy. Fat calories slow metabolism.

Most of the energy fat provides is stored in the waist, hips, thighs, and buttocks. Your body doesn't know when you are going to eat again, so it behaves as if every meal were its last. Whatever extra energy your body can find is stored in the form of fat.

The Most Dangerous Calorie

Food contains energy and the amount of energy a food contains can be measured in calories. A pound of fat contains 3,500 calories. Scientists formerly thought that consuming 3,500 calories more than the body needed would result in gaining a pound of fat. Conversely, eating 3,500 fewer calories than the body needed would "burn" that many calories from the stored fat, resulting in the loss of a pound.

In other words, researchers thought *the source* of calories didn't matter. A calorie from a piece of cake was no different than a calorie from a carrot. However, this is not true.

The most dangerous calorie is a fat calorie. *Fat calories are fattening.* Wherever you see the most fat on your body right now is exactly where your fat will continue to be deposited. Eat a fat, rich dessert—like apple pie with ice cream—and it will apply itself directly to your fattest spots.

When fat is consumed, the process of turning it into body fat is simple. Eat 100 calories of dietary fat, like butter, and you can expect 97 of them to end up on your hips, thighs, and stomach—somewhere on you. In contrast, your body must burn 23 calories to turn 100 calories of carbohydrates into body fat.

Keys to Weight Control

Fat cells, once created, will never go away. But you can outsmart your fat cells! With proper diet and exercise, a person can draw stored energy from the fat cells and reduce their size. But the cell itself will always remain.

You can outsmart your fat cells by not eating large amounts of food once you have lost the desired weight. Overeating signals the body to store fat and causes fat cells to divide. Avoid eating binges where you might eat six donuts or a quart of ice cream.

For example, if you were traveling and did not stop for breakfast or lunch, you might be famished by dinner. You may think you can afford to eat more since you had missed eating all day. But eating a large amount at one time could trigger your body into making more fat cells.

Another key to weight control is to substitute complex carbohydrates for fat. When you do, you can eat without fear of everything turning into fat. But in turning to carbohydrates a person must still use caution. For example, pasta is great until you put a rich, fat, creamy sauce on it. Rice is good, but leave the gravy in the bowl.

If you find after you switch to a low-fat, high-carbohydrate diet that you are hungry all the time and never feel full, try eating several small meals a day instead of three large meals. Eating this way will hinder the brain from giving its hormonal signal that you are hungry.

Praising Pasta

Energy found in complex carbohydrates such as pasta, fresh fruits, and vegetables is stored in small amounts in the muscles and the liver in the form of glycogen. Under normal circumstances glycogen never turns to fat. I have always said, "If you have to overeat, overeat on complex carbohydrates."

Spaghetti is a good example of what a high complex carbohydrate can do for you. Do you think spaghetti has the same potential as steak for making you fat? Scientists say it doesn't.

In a controlled study, a group of prison volunteers were overfed until they were classified obese. These formerly lean men were divided into two groups: one group received a high-fat diet while the other was fed a high-carbohydrate diet. Those overfed on the high-carbohydrate diet gained weight with great difficulty while those overfed on fat foods gained rapidly.

Your body uses a higher percentage of energy to convert carbohydrates into body fat than it does to convert dietary fat into body fat. Compare the different ways your metabolism handles spaghetti and steak. Twenty-five percent of the calories in a cup of spaghetti are used in getting the food ready for storage. With steak, only 3 percent of the calories are burned and the balance is stored. A wise dieter will eat carbohydrates that burn calories in the process of digestion.

Fats Vs. Carbohydrates

A high-carbohydrate diet seems to stimulate your body's metabolism in much the same way that exercise does—causing you to burn more calories while at the same time enabling you to maintain high energy at a lower body weight. Such a diet also helps you feel full and satisfied so you won't overeat.

You must feel satisfied in order to know when to stop eating. Have you ever noticed that eating a meal high in fat leaves you hungry again a couple of hours later? For example, a hot dog, potato chips, and a cupcake might satisfy you for an hour or two, but hunger pangs soon return.

In contrast, a meal of spaghetti, pita bread, and fruit will leave you feeling satisfied. Complex carbohydrates keep you from overeating. You can't eat a bag of apples—just a few will satisfy the average person. But simple carbohydrates, like sweet desserts, can be consumed in huge quantities without providing satisfaction. In fact, some people can eat a whole cake or a quart of ice cream and still feel dissatisfied.

Carbohydrates affect the body's insulin and signal when we are full. Carbohydrates stimulate insulin. Fats do not. This is why you feel full after eating pasta, a baked potato, vegetables, bread or fruit. All these foods affect the insulin level in your body.

Our bodies are programmed to store fat in order to survive. Should we be deprived of food for any length of time, the body has the capacity to live off the stored energy of fat for as long as two or three months if necessary.

In contrast, carbohydrates that are not burned for fuel are turned into glycogen. Only one-half to one pound of glycogen can be stored in the muscles and liver. The remainder is passed off as waste material. A system of checks and balances goes into effect when we eat complex carbo-hydrates that help the body maintain steady weight. With fats, however, no such system exists. In fact, the metabolic system is not even triggered by fats because fats do not stimulate insulin.

Carbohydrates speed up the metabolism because they must go through a more complicated process of digestion and storage. This results in a much greater loss of heat and stimulating the heart and all body processes.

How To Stop Snacking Between Meals

Americans want instant everything. Too many of us have never learned that slowing down and taking time to enjoy each moment is the only way to reduce stress and enhance life. We gobble down fat-saturated burgers and fries, barely tasting them in order to "instantly" satisfy hunger. We hardly know we've eaten. No wonder hunger pains return in less than an hour.

How much better to smell a tasty, nutritious meal as it is cooked. We need to enjoy relaxing meals with our family or friends. When we take time to chew and enjoy our food, our brain has time to get the news across to our entire body that it has just been fed and satisfied. Snacking to curb hunger twinges thirty minutes later doesn't occur because the body has been fully satisfied.

Studies have shown that obese persons many times do not even taste what is in their mouth. They tend to just hastily shovel it in—thinking only of the next mouthful. Slow down if you are guilty of this and take time to enjoy each bite. You will find yourself eating less and being satisfied sooner.

The Flavor Factor

Let's pretend that for weeks now you have faithfully fol-lowed your diet of low-fat, low-calorie foods. Just as the scales are tipping in your favor, you are seized with an uncontrollable urge to eat pizza, potato chips—anything with flavor.

Are you just a weak-willed, lily liver? No, you are perfectly normal. New research tells us that flavor may be critical to the success of any weight-loss diet. Depriving your senses of taste and smell with bland, boring foods could put your diet on the "critical list."

Why is flavor so important? Odors and tastes are wired to the limbic system, the "pleasure centers" of the brain. When food touches the tongue, your taste buds go to work on the four basic flavors—bitter, sweet, salty, and sour. Chewing also forces odors up the back of the throat and into the nose, which stimulates your sense of smell and intensifies the food's taste.

Flavor also affects us psychologically. We often associate flavors with pleasant or unpleasant memories. Think of the memories that well up in your mind when you bite into a fresh-baked cookie that tastes like the ones Mom used to bake.

We all have the need for a certain amount of flavor in our food. Until we reach our flavor set point, we tend to keep eating. Research tells us that overweight people have a higher flavor set point than people of average weight.

Overweight people were tested to see if they would eat less food if they had more flavor. Three groups were tested. In two groups the food was sprayed with a flavor enhancer that made tuna taste tunaier and macaroni and cheese taste cheesier. The groups using the flavor enhancer lost more weight. Flavor can make a difference to the dieter.

Re-adjusting Your Taste Buds

So how do you tackle the flavor problem when you want to lose weight? Start by eating a variety of foods at every meal and never eat two consecutive bites of the same food.

Your senses of taste and smell tire when they are overloaded with the same flavor.

Chew your food well to release more of the flavor and smell. Heating your food, which releases more of the aroma, may satisfy your taste buds sooner so you eat less. Some low-calorie foods such as tuna or cauliflower taste better cold, however.

The best course of action is to allow your body and your taste buds time to adjust to the flavor of less fattening foods. In time you will actually prefer the taste of carbohydrates. One day you'll realize, "Hey, I really would rather have an apple than a Twinkie!"

Fat foods taste better and give you more of a feeling of fullness than carbohydrates, especially until you get used to the flavor of less fattening foods. Why doesn't sherbet taste as good and satisfying as ice cream? Both desserts are cold, sweet, and refreshing, yet ice cream satisfies the hunger so much better.

The answer is fat. Ice cream has lots of fat. Sherbet has very little. According to scientists, fat carries the flavor of a food. Most of a food's flavor is carried in its aroma, and most odor molecules dissolve only in fat. That's why the more fattening a food is, the better it smells. And the better it smells, the better it tastes.

The key to losing weight is to satisfy the love-of-fat-tastes without eating the fat. Studies have shown that in many cases, what an obese person is craving is the flavor of fattening foods rather than the foods themselves. When deprived of this flavor, they often become depressed and discouraged with a diet.

Don't Be a Pie Baby

Have you ever walked through a cafeteria and noticed the group of ladies holding up the line trying to decide which piece of pie they should have for dessert? I have nicknamed these people "pie babies." Selecting the right piece of pie is the biggest decision of the day for some of them.

Through my quest for personal health and vitality, my research has clearly shown me that these desserts have absolutely no nutrition to offer my body—just empty calories that are deposited in my fat cells.

I used to say, "If you don't want to look like a Big Mac, don't eat a Big Mac," and I really believe that. I don't want to be a "pie baby." I want to have lots of energy. Fruit is the only kind of dessert I have come to enjoy. I know fat is sugar's best friend, and it's the fat in desserts that steals away my health and robs me of the nutrients I need. Say *no* to becoming a "pie baby."

You might say, "Well, I only had a tiny piece of pecan pie today." That little piece was probably at least 900 calories. We don't need much more than 900 calories in an entire day! At my age 1200 calories is about all I can eat during a day. A little piece of pie can do you in because 80 percent of it will be stored as fat on your body. Learn to think of your body being a very efficient engine that needs quality fuel.

Time Off For Good Behavior?

"I bet you don't eat at all to stay so slim," people have told me. I do enjoy eating, and I eat on a regular basis. My built-in clock tells me when it's time to eat, and I stick to that schedule.

Having learned that fat foods make me fat, I simply avoid them like the plague. I don't eat fried foods, sweets, or foods that are loaded with fat. I keep seeing that sign in my mind, "The fat you eat is the fat you will wear." It's true.

I used to eat very carefully all week and then indulge in my favorite foods on weekends—fried chicken, desserts— whatever I wanted. After strictly adhering to my diet, it was easy to rationalize a weekend splurge. This behavior caught up with me eventually. Unless you want to have a weight problem and be unhealthy for the rest of your life, learn to eat properly seven days a week.

Remember, your eating should glorify God. Eating healthy is like the Christian lifestyle—we don't get days off for good behavior. Every day we are to glorify God in every area of our lives. See your enemy—the villain is *fat*. Learn where it is hiding in food so you can avoid it.

5

Losing Weight the Sensible Way

Is your weight a matter of destiny or determination? Has your size more or less been pre-determined by heredity?

A woman once asked her doctor if she should work hard to lose weight or just give up since both her parents were obese. Having read that obesity is inherited, she wondered if she should even try to lose weight.

While we inherit the *tendency* to be a certain size, through sensible eating and exercise we can control much of what nature has given us. According to scientific studies, even an adopted child will resemble his or her natural parents in weight. One's fat distribution points and body shape are inherited as well as the propagation, accumulation, and number of fat cells.

Your excess fat is destined to be stored in much the same places as it is on your parents' bodies. If your mother is over-weight and her heaviest accumulation of fat is in her hips, then that is most likely where yours would be if you were overweight.

But here's the good news! Just because one or both of your parents were obese, you do not have to be. Your fat cells may have inherited the tendency to divide and multiply rapidly, but you can determine their destiny. Through proper eating and exercise, you have the ability to greatly modify what nature has given you.

Participate in controlling your health. You must believe that you have the ability to determine your shape just as you have the ability to control how you look through hairstyle and make-up.

For example, take a person who wears glasses and has pale skin, small eyes, a long nose, and lifeless hair. With contacts for her eyes, make-up for her face, highlights for her hair, and possibly a perm, she can be a very attractive person. *You* can control to a great extent what nature has given you and even modify it for your own good.

Personalized Weight Loss

Some people were never meant to be pencil thin. New studies have shown that 80 percent of the variations of body weight are determined by heredity.

I am not saying that some people were meant to be obese. Certainly not! But moderate amounts of weight gained by some women in the hips and thighs during puberty and pregnancies may be just what nature programmed for their bodies.

For some people, going on an 800-calorie diet merely signals their bodies to resist starvation and frantically store fat. Such a person can lose more on a sensible 1200-1400 calorie diet combined with exercise.

A genetic predisposition toward being overweight, a larger number of fat cells, long-established habits of overeating, and lack of exercise are reasons for having difficulty in reaching your ideal weight. If you weigh more than the weight tables say you should, don't be discouraged. Those tables do not take into account other factors, including how your weight is distributed.

Why starve yourself down to what a table says is your ideal weight, if you have to continue to starve to stay there? More important than what you weigh is how good you feel at a particular weight. In other words, be yourself. Your ideal weight should be what feels and looks best on you.

Maintaining Your Correct Weight

Many doctors do not place much stock in traditional height and weight tables. The charts have been found to be right for people around forty years of age, but too liberal for young adults and too restrictive for older people. In other words, twenty-year-olds should weigh less and sixty-year-olds should be allowed to weigh more than the charts indicate.

To maintain your correct weight, multiply the weight times fifteen. This will give you the total calories you can take in and still maintain the weight. If you don't exercise any given day, subtract 300 calories from the total number of calories you can consume.

Here's how this formula works. Suppose a woman weighing 100 pounds wants to maintain that weight. Using this formula she calculates 100 X 15 or 1500 calories that she may eat each day if she exercises for at least thirty minutes. If she doesn't exercise, she must subtract 300 calories from 1500 and consume only 1200 calories that day.

Keep track of your calorie intake each day. A calorie counter is a worthwhile purchase for the person serious about maintaining a correct weight. These are usually available in supermarkets and variety stores. Keep it with you at all times, and memorize the calorie content of foods.

How to Keep the Fat Off

Research has proven the importance of exercise in the quest for weight loss. One particular study focused on a group of forty-two women who were at least twenty pounds overweight with a body fat content of 41 percent. These women were measured before an exercise-diet program began and again after each five-pound weight loss.

As the fat began to come off, a pattern of weight loss emerged. With each woman the first fat loss was in the waist and mid-section. After ten pounds were lost, the subjects began losing in waist, thighs, buttocks, and upper arms. Total muscle mass increased by one pound.

After the loss of fifteen pounds, reduction continued in all areas mentioned with the buttocks showing the greatest loss. By this time the women had lost an average of 12.3 inches. After a twenty-pound loss, the body had changed all over and reduction had occurred in all the problem areas. In the end the amount of fat lost from the trunk region of the body was twice that lost in the extremities (face, hands, and feet).

The biggest pay-off came by sticking to the program. The ten-pound loss produced twice the reduction in measurement of the five-pound loss. A twenty-pound loss resulted in three times the reductions of the ten-pound loss.

What happens when people diet to the exclusion of exercise? The results from a study of long-distance runners proves that exercise is necessary to keeping fat down. The runners were divided into two groups: one group continued to train after the marathon; another stopped all training. Even though the group that stopped training continued to eat a low-fat diet, they re-gained 95 percent of their pre-training fat. Those who continued in training maintained their ideal weight.

Don't Give Up

People often get discouraged and quit exercising because they don't see dramatic, fast results like someone else who follows the same regimen. Others have asked me, "Some people eat more than I, but they don't gain weight. Why?"

Losing or gaining weight is greatly determined by the balance between energy input (food and drink) and energy output (loss of heat energy due to metabolic response to food and exercise). Since energy output differs from person to person so does weight loss.

Not only does your metabolic rate differ from that of others but your own rate can change within a period of a few weeks. What causes this? Hormonal changes, emotional stress, nutrition, and many other factors can alter metabolism. Many people blame thyroid problems for weight gain. In reality, however, thyroid malfunction affects only about 2 percent of the overweight population.

If your metabolism makes weight loss unusually difficult, don't give up and don't be discouraged. Never compare your progress with others. Fat, like melting snow, is going to be hardest to lose where it is highest and deepest. Never expect overnight "anything" when it comes to losing weight. The only thing you can lose overnight or in a week is water weight.

Each body is different, and how we respond to diet and exercise is to a great extent controlled by genetics. Some people may be able to burn fat faster than others, depending on fat-cell size and individual metabolism. In any case, exercise is necessary in order to increase your body's metabolism so that it burns energy at its optimum rate.

But I Hate To Exercise

Recent studies have shown that exercise does not have to be hard to be good. In fact, the more pleasant exercise is for you, the more good it does you. Trying to do too much too soon will only discourage you. Attempting to carry out an exercise program designed for athletes or aerobics specialists may tempt you to give up before you derive any physical benefits. Exercise should feel natural and should be one of the highlights of your day.

Let me explode one myth that may be keeping you from a healthier life. Exercise does not have to be torture.

In fact, pain is a warning that the body is being overly stressed. If you experience pain while exercising, slack off and try something less stressful.

Exercise should be vigorous enough to get the heart pumping but should not deplete you of your strength. You need not fear exercising until the perspiration appears. Perspiration is a sign that your heart is being exercised. If you begin to drip with perspiration, however, you may be pushing yourself too far.

More important than the degree of exercise is the regularity. The best exercise allows you to stay within your own personal limits and should be convenient for you to do at least three times a week for thirty to forty-five minutes. I still prefer a more consistent program of exercising at least six days a week.

Gaining Weight with Age

People may protest, "I don't eat anymore than I always have, yet I continue to gain weight. Why?"

I believe them. Eating is not their problem but lack of exercise probably is, especially if they are between the ages of twenty-five and fifty-five. What gradually happens to our bodies parallels what happens to a broken arm when it is put into a cast for several weeks. The muscles seem to "atrophy" or waste away due to the immobility of the arm.

When people over the age of twenty-five do not exercise regularly, they can lose lean muscle mass—around fifteen pounds of it—due to inactivity. A person may weigh the same at fifty-five as he did at twenty-five but with fifteen pounds less lean muscle and fifteen pounds more fat on him. Because most of us gain one pound per year after the age of twenty-five no matter what, you can see how easy it is to gain forty-five pounds of fat by age fifty-five with no significant changes in diet or food intake.

The key to weight control is regular and vigorous exercise. Exercise will not only help burn up the calories we consume but will also help keep them from being stored as fat. The careful, wise eater will not only lose weight consistently but will have a firmer, stronger body to boot.

The Dieter's Stalemate

Another frequent question I am asked is, "Why do I lose weight to a certain point and then stop losing even though I continue with my diet?"

Your body's metabolism slows down with dieting. Why? Any weight loss improves the body's efficiency. You will require less energy and burn fewer calories at a lower weight. For instance, a woman weighing 180 pounds uses more energy to vacuum the floor than she would at 150 pounds.

So how can you keep losing weight once you hit the stalemate? Increase your exercise.

Failure to preserve muscle mass is a serious flaw in most diets. Too many dieters prefer a low-calorie diet with no exercise. This imbalanced approach to weight loss just won't get the job done. Some studies suggest a 7 percent increase in physical exercise for every ten-pound loss. Lean muscle mass increases with exercise and so does metabolism and the burning of calories.

Your basal metabolic rate (the amount of energy used while at rest) is determined by the amount of lean muscle you have. An unsupervised or very low-calorie fad diet causes you to lose lean muscle mass and lowers your basal metabolic rate. During a diet, your body requires fewer calories at rest and during exercise. Over a period of time, this causes weight gain even if you are eating fewer calories.

Fat Trapping

Dieting causes your body to lose its ability to shed fat and leads to a very dangerous increase in body fat percentage. As you continue with a low-fat diet and no exercise, you lose lean muscle mass and slowly build up fat all over your body.

All diets can produce weight loss, but all weight loss is not equal. Remember, the perfect diet results in maximum fat loss and minimum lean muscle loss. This is what happens when you follow a sensible eating plan and exercise. You burn fat and maintain your lean muscle mass.

Digestion burns calories. If you go for a walk fifteen minutes after a meal, you burn a lot of calories before they have the chance to be stored as fat. If you do this after each meal, you will be way ahead of the game. You can speed up your metabolism by as much as 20 percent.

If, however, you relax in a chair after dinner, most of the calories you've just consumed will be stored as fat. Your body just packs those calories away in fat cells, and you wear them to work the next day.

Battle The Fat, Not the Scales

Doctors warn that today's preoccupation with thinness can be harmful. Some people who do not need to lose weight are pushing themselves to the breaking point. Resist the destructive temptation to judge your looks and your self-worth by what you read on the scale and see in magazines and on TV. In fact, stay away from the scales as much as possible while dieting.

A preoccupation with your size can lead to anorexia and other eating disorders. Just concentrate on a healthy low-fat diet and an exercise program you can live with, and forget the scales. Next thing you know, you will be looking at a more slender, healthy you.

The right way to check weight loss is to measure your waist, hips, and thighs once a week. This records fat loss more precisely. The scales are not always accurate because weight loss can occur with loss of fluid or lean muscle mass. A tape measure reveals fat loss while the scale could be showing a loss of fluid, lean muscle mass, or fat. Remember, it's fat you want to lose.

Tips On Attitude

Don't let dieting and exercise control your life so that you think of nothing else. Take time to enjoy life—explore nature, take up a hobby, read a good book. Think on good things and don't just live for yourself. Love and serve others as Christ has set the example before you.

Don't let your battle with food steal your peace and joy.

> Do not be anxious about anything, but in everything, by prayer and petition, with thanksgiving, present your requests to God. And the peace of God, which transcends all understanding, will guard your hearts and your minds in Christ Jesus—Philippians 4:6,7, NIV.

Lean on the Lord and keep your eyes on Him. He's on your side and if you do your part, He will take care of the rest. The Lord wants you to be healthy and fit. He will provide the strength and help you need to become the best person you can be in Him. When you exercise or go for a walk, begin to thank the Lord for each block you walk. Thank the Lord for every exercise you can do.

When I look at food now, I ask, "What is this going to do for me? Will this help me glorify God in my body?"

I urge you, if you are overweight, resolve now to shed those unnecessary pounds with God's help.

> Therefore, since we are surrounded by such a great cloud of witnesses, let us throw off everything that hinders and the sin that so easily entangles, and let us run with perseverence the race marked out for us—Hebrews 12:1, NIV.

How to Get Started

Two questions are often asked by the beginning dieter. The first is, "When is the best time to begin a weight loss program?" The second is, "What can you do when you 'fall off the wagon'?"

To answer the first—the best time to begin dieting is probably at the beginning of the year or a month, or when your medical condition frightens you into it. The worst time is when you need to fit into a dress for a wedding in three weeks. That kind of crash dieting leads you into the yo-yo syndrome where you will lose fat and muscle but will regain only fat. On such a diet your potential for easy regain of body fat increases while your ability to burn calories steadily decreases.

Get your doctor's approval before starting any diet. Make sure you're providing your body with all its essential nutrients. And *never* take in less than 1,000 calories per day. There is no way you can maintain a balanced diet on anything below this.

This may be a good place to plead with you to never think fluid pills are the answer to weight loss. If you are truly bothered with fluid build-up, drinking lots of water is the best way to get rid of the excess fluid. If you drink six to ten glasses of water each day, you will soon begin to see that fluid retention is less and less of a problem with you. You will be trotting to the bathroom more, but that's okay.

Looking at a thinner you in the mirror is great. Even better are the decreased cholesterol and triglyceride levels when you follow a low-fat way of eating and a daily exercise plan. When blood fat levels go down, so does your risk of heart attack.

What do you do when you fall off the wagon? First, don't feel guilty. You will only eat more. People make the mistake of thinking of a diet as a sort of "ritual" and if they break their routine, they develop a sense of guilt and shame.

This lowers self-esteem and can undermine almost any weight loss program. Every day is a new day. Overindulging at one meal will not make you fat. If you fail one day, just begin again the next day.

Losing weight this way is slow, but it works and it lasts. If you slip and overeat, compensate by doubling up on the exercise. No magic pill or potion exists for losing weight. Face that fact and get on with the business of getting into shape.

6

Dangerous Dieting

The nation's number one obsession and frustration seems to be the pursuit of a slender body. Approximately 90 percent of Americans think they weigh too much, according to a 1986 survey by *Better Homes and Gardens*.

This preoccupation with slimness is at once both sad and humorous. Some 1985 figures showed that Americans spent five billion dollars on battling their bulges. You can rest assured that most of that money was wasted on useless fad diets, pills, and books. Those who fall for the quick weight-loss gimmicks are just getting thinner wallets not thinner bodies.

Appetite suppressants, diuretics, and laxatives are the medications many people look to for a "quick fix" for their weight problems. No matter what you see in advertising, there are no quick fixes for weight control. Sudden weight loss, like the inheritance quickly gained at the beginning, will not be blessed in the end. (See Proverbs 20:21, NIV).

Losing weight simply means eating right and exercising. If you stick to a good program, you will lose weight. There are no short cuts or miracle cures. Remember, slow losers do lose; it may take longer but the weight also stays off.

The Dangers of Diet Aids

Not only are over-the-counter diet aids useless for long-term weight control, they are dangerous and can even be deadly. Some diet pills, when taken with alcohol or caffeine, can aggravate already existing high blood pressure and heart conditions. That dangerous combination may even lead to coma or death.

Some users of diet aids have suffered damage to the nervous system, personality changes, permanent deformities, and even death from cerebral bleeding. The very chemicals in these aids that suppress the appetite also stimulate the nervous system, speed up heart rate, raise blood pressure, and cause spasms of blood vessels in the brain.

Normal, healthy people with no previous history of hypertension have taken diet aids and developed bleeding of the brain that resulted in death. Caffeine, which is often added to diet pills, only enhances the problem. Even if you take caffeine-free diet pills, but you consume caffeinated drinks such as coffee, tea, and most carbonated beverages, the dangers remain. Teens and children can purchase diet pills and take them without any adult supervision. Due to their ready availability over the counter, this makes diet pills doubly dangerous.

Diuretics or water pills can wipe you out physically. Diuretics only relieve you of water weight that is easily regained after the pill wears off. Since many diuretics contain caffeine, the problem of hypertension also exists. Diuretics are even a threat to your kidneys because of the ammonium chloride they contain.

Laxatives only succeed in helping you lose water weight at the risk of causing dehydration and addiction. When abused, laxatives can permanently disrupt normal functioning of the bowels. A person can become so dependant on laxatives, they cannot have a bowel movement without them.

Dangerous Dieting

Before we look at safe, sensible weight loss, I want to discuss dangerous dieting with you. Trading calories for weight loss may be costly to your emotional and physical health.

Healthy, overweight men who decreased their food intake from 3,000 to 1,500 calories per day experienced all kinds of health problems at the end of six months. They suffered depression, anemia, edema, slowing of heartbeat, fatigue, and lack of endurance.

Any diet that relies heavily on one food, such as grapefruit, is damaging to your health. Low-calorie, liquid diets can be deadly. I know of one man who developed cancer of the lymph glands within six months after going on a popular, low-calorie liquid diet. He firmly believes, and his doctors agree (although there is no way to scientifically prove it), that the diet triggered a chemical imbalance within his body that caused the cancer growth to occur.

The Low-Carbohydrate Diet

One of the most dangerous diets is a low-carbohydrate diet. You may lose weight on such a regimen, but it's mostly water and other body fluids—not fat. As soon as you come off that diet, the water weight quickly returns.

One doctor reports that a patient gained twenty pounds of water weight in one weekend immediately after going off a low-calorie crash diet. Low-carbohydrate diets are either high-protein or high-fat or both. Since both fats and proteins need the glucose that carbohydrates provide in order to be metabolized, where can all those unburned calories go except in storage?

A low-carbohydrate diet can lead to all kinds of health problems: gout, irregular heartbeats, fatigue, blood pressure abnormalities, dehydration, kidney malfunction, and high cholesterol.

Expectant mothers must *never* try this diet. A baby's nervous system can only metabolize glucose for energy. If the supply of glucose is shut off for even a short time, damage can occur to the baby.

Dieting Doomed to Fail

An article I read recently stated that love may be better the second time around, but when it comes to fat, you had better forget it. Few things in life are more discouraging than regaining weight you fought so hard to lose.

Did you know that crash dieting makes you gain more weight? Tests with laboratory animals and people have clearly shown that each time you go on a crash diet to lose weight, it takes longer to shed the weight and it becomes easier to regain.

Why does crash dieting make it harder to lose weight? Every time we go on a crash diet, we lose muscle and fat. When we resume our high-fat diets that made us overweight in the first place, we regain mostly fat.

With each crash diet, you become "fatter." You slowly lose muscle with dieting, and when you start regaining you put fat on. Crash dieting causes loss of lean muscle mass. Muscles burn calories. Each time you crash diet, you have less muscle available to burn fat. The result? Crash dieters inevitably just get fatter.

Crash Dieting

A hormonal factor also makes it more difficult to lose weight on low-calorie diets. When you eat fewer than 800 calories a day, your thyroid gland produces less T-3, which is a hormone that regulates your metabolic rate. This, in turn, temporarily reduces your metabolic rate by about 15 percent.

Once you eat a normal diet, your T-3 level returns to normal. But because you've lost muscle mass in the process, your metabolic rate is lower than before you started the low-calorie diet. As a result, fewer calories are burned.

You can reverse a sluggish metabolism by eating right and exercising, which will build up your muscle mass. Remember, the muscles are the motors of the body and the fat goes along for the ride.

Crash dieting is a triple threat to permanent weight loss because:

1. You lower your T-3 level and reduce your calorie-burning power as you diet.
2. You lose lean muscle mass. When you reduce muscle, you reduce your body's ability to burn calories.
3. You regain mostly fat when you return to your old way of eating so repeated crash dieting makes you fatter by increasing your fat-to-muscle mass.

My advice—if you are not exercising, begin today. Walk as briskly as you can for thirty minutes each day. This will build up your lean muscle mass and give you energy. Follow a diet that is not over 30 percent fat, about 15 percent protein, and the balance in complex carbohydrates (fruits, vegetables, and whole grains like rice, bread, pasta, and cereals). You will have more energy and feel so much better.

The Yo-Yo Syndrome

Do you diet and lose weight only to put it right back on? If you've ever said, "No problem! I'll just diet again," you probably don't realize what you're doing to yourself. Repeated dieting sets your body into a pattern of loss and quick regain.

Severely lowering your caloric intake mimics starvation, which forces your body to conserve energy, lower its metabolic rate, and store every calorie it can grab as fat.

With each diet and regain you go through, it becomes harder and harder to lose what is regained and easier and easier to regain what few pounds you do lose.

This loss and regain pattern leads to hypertension and bigger bodies in the long run. Tests on people and animals show that an endless cycle of dieting, starving, and binging may be triggered.

Studies with laboratory animals who were placed on the equivalent of human crash diets showed weight loss among the animals. But as soon as they were allowed to eat freely again, they quickly regained the lost weight and became heavier than they had been prior to the diet. Why? What they regained was all fat and no lean muscle tissue. This is why exercise is so important with a diet.

When I lost 20 percent of my body weight through stress at age twenty-seven, the weight I lost was lean muscle mass. Once I started regaining weight, I noticed that my clothes didn't fit! This time when I weighed 100 pounds, I was two sizes bigger in the hips and thighs. What happened?

My muscles had wasted away because I didn't exercise in conjunction with my initial weight loss or the subsequent weight gain. I had lost lean muscle mass but had replaced it with fat. That's why exercise is important for us at all times—whether we are losing weight, putting some weight back on, or just maintaining our bodies. Daily exercise helps retain muscle mass, and it burns fat.

Studies have been conducted with laboratory animals and people that show that yo-yo dieting can:

1. Increase the proportion of fat to lean tissue.
2. Redistribute body fat, shifting it from the hips and thighs to the abdomen, which is very dangerous to your health.
3. Increase the desire for fatty foods.
4. Increase the risk of heart disease.
5. Seriously distort your body's weight-regulation system.

In studies where people lost 10 percent of their body weight, they reduced risk of coronary heart disease by 20 percent. When these same people regained 10 percent of their body weight, they raised their risk by 30 percent. That means if your weight drops from 150 to 135 pounds and then creeps back to 150 again, you are left with a higher risk of heart disease than before dieting began.

Dieting has to be taken seriously. You have to make up your mind when you lose weight that you are not going to put it back on. If you do, you increase your risk of disease. Dieting is nothing to play around with.

Dieting or Starving?

When you cut calories, your body slows its basal metabolic rate. Your body cannot tell the difference between a diet and starvation. If you were starving, your body would cut the calories it burns. Unfortunately, your body responds the same way to a diet, but a lowered metabolism doesn't help you lose weight. That's why you reach a frustrating plateau where you can't seem to lose any additional weight. Your slowed metabolism is working against your diet.

After repeated yo-yo dieting, more severe calorie restrictions and more time were required to achieve the same weight loss. The researchers saw this with the laboratory rats. The yo-yo dieting cycles messed up their metabolisms. On the first diet it took the rats forty-five days to become obese. On the second bout of dieting, it took only fourteen days for the rats to become obese.

Other studies reveal even more disturbing news about crash diets. Extremely low-calorie diets will trigger the body to protect the brain cells and fat cells. Guess what is used for energy? Your lean muscle cells.

Some people have literally starved themselves to death. When autopsies were performed on their bodies, pathologists discovered that the body had been living off of itself!

Sometimes part of a heart or other vital organ was eaten away by the body itself. If a diet is well-balanced and if the person exercises, the weight loss will be fat, and vital muscle tissue will not be attacked.

Changing Your Set Point

A woman wrote her doctor that she was desperately trying to lose weight and was only eating one meal a day. But she couldn't seem to get past a certain point. Did he have any suggestions? The doctor replied, "Yes, start eating." Why would he say that?

Crash diets at first bring a drastic decrease in body weight but most of it comes from muscle and water loss—not fat. The weight is quickly and easily regained once the diet ends.

The brain has a Weight Regulating Mechanism (WRM) that chooses the amount of fat it considers ideal for your body. The fat level chosen by the WRM is called the "set point." Your set point is determined by genetics, food intake, and exercising habits.

This set point is similar to your home thermostat that kicks on the furnace when the temperature falls. A raised set point stimulates the hunger drive and conserves energy. A lower set point suppresses the hunger drive and improves the fat-burning process.

WRM controls body weight in two critically important ways. First, it influences the amount of food you eat, increasing or decreasing your appetite as needed to maintain your set point. Second, it can trigger systems in the body to waste excess energy if you overeat or to conserve energy if you eat too little.

Your Set Point and Metabolism

Irregular eating habits force the body to conserve energy. Cutting back drastically on food or skipping a meal alerts the WRM, which immediately slows the body's metabolism. Each time you eat, enzymes are secreted in the stomach that increase your metabolism. Regular eating habits cause frequent secretions of these enzymes.

The body speeds up metabolism when meals come regularly. Knowing there is no need to store fat because food is coming in on schedule, your body becomes more efficient at burning fat. If, however, you have been yo-yoing with your diet, it will take time to re-adjust your thermostat.

The body's desire to protect against starvation explains why people will lose a little at first and then just stop. The brain doesn't know that you are just going on a temporary crash diet. A starvation reading causes your body to shut down all unnecessary energy expenditure to protect itself. Even on the best diet, metabolism may slow to a crawl. If you're lying in bed not moving, you will burn sixty calories per hour. If you're on a diet, however, you will burn only fifty. By increasing your metabolism with exercise, you will burn seventy calories per hour. Exercise will get you past the stalemate that is brought on by the brain's reaction to starvation signals.

Nibbling vs. Belly Busters

When a dieter ends his low-calorie regimen and returns to normal eating, he must be sure to remain on a low-fat, high complex carbohydrate diet, avoiding fats and sweets. He must avoid eating large portions to prevent the formation of new fat cells.

Nibbling six small meals a day is preferable to filling up on three huge ones. Your behavior and your attitude will have a lot to do with whether you keep your weight off once you lose it.

Experiments with laboratory animals show that several small meals a day will keep the body from storing as much fat. Eating two large meals a day causes the stomach and intestines to enlarge to accommodate this large influx of food. With the small intestine enlarged to handle the food, the body absorbs calories at a much greater rate because large amounts of insulin must be released to help process this influx.

One of insulin's jobs is to put fat into storage. Nibbling on several small meals a day is preferable to eating three belly busters. For those trying to lose weight, three large meals a day encourages fat storage.

Burning Up Those Calories

Weight loss can be explained in one word—heat. Calorie burning more than calorie counting is the key to successful weight loss and maintenance. The heat the body generates when we eat is called thermogenesis. This heat burns up calories that would otherwise end up being stored as fat.

Lean muscle build-up, not fat loss, is most responsible for increasing the body's metabolism. The more muscle, the greater the metabolic burning of calories. Most diets fail to keep weight off because they result in a loss of lean muscle as well as fat. This reduces your calorie-burning power, leaving you "fatter." A diet high in complex carbohydrates and exercise causes you to lose fat, not muscle.

We can maximize heat production in three areas:

1. Resting metabolic rate (the number of calories burned for normal body functions— approximately 60 percent of calories).
2. Physical activity (burns about 25 percent).
3. Thermic effect of food (burns about 15 percent).

When you cut calories, you cut your metabolic rate or, in other words, burn fewer calories to produce less heat. You may decrease your metabolism by as much as 15 to 30 percent by dieting.

You can burn up to 300 calories a day just by eating the right foods. Carbohydrates and protein are hot burners; fat is not. When you consume 200 calories worth of fat, only 3 percent of this amount is burned (six calories), which leaves 194 calories for storage on the body.

Diet alone won't keep you slim. Aerobic exercise kicks up your metabolism by 10 to 15 percent. Exercise ensures you lose the right kind of weight—fat not lean muscle mass. In a study of exercisers versus non-exercisers, in an 18-pound loss, 11 pounds of fat and 7 pounds of muscle were lost on the non-exerciser. The exerciser lost 23 pounds of fat and gained 4 pounds of muscle. The exerciser lost weight and boosted metabolism.

Dieting Can Make You Happy

Repeat after me, "I'm dieting, and I'm in a good mood." Just can't get the words out? I don't blame you. Not many people feel that way about their diets. But new evidence reveals that shedding pounds sensibly can be a real mood booster especially when we start changing our behavior.

Studies in the 1960s revealed that dieters tended to become anxious and depressed. This depression comes about when a person is on a low-calorie, unbalanced diet. More recent studies show that once the pounds begin to come off the mood improves if a diet is balanced and not too low calorically.

In one study a group of seventy-six men and women were put on a moderate weight loss program designed to pare off two pounds per week. Their daily food intake totaled 1,200 calories for women and 1,500 calories for men. They could eat what they wanted from a well-balanced diet that was low in fat, high in complex carbohydrates, and moderate in protein, but had to stay within their calorie count.

They also attended weekly hour-long behavior modification meetings led by a psychologist and nutritionist.

They learned how to set goals and eat only when hungry. At the end of ten weeks, the dieters lost an average of 12.2 pounds, and their moods improved as their weight went down.

I used to drastically cut back on my food intake to lose weight. Breakfast and lunch were no problem, but I frequently gorged myself on dinner. If I ate like a bird for several days, and then the bottom dropped out of my self-control, I absolutely stuffed myself.

Cutting back on my calorie intake seemed to affect my moods. I got cross and snapped at my friends. Over the years I've discovered cutting back drastically on calories is unwise. Now I lower my fat intake but eat enough good foods like fruits, vegetables, and whole grains.

If You Need Motivation

I recently read an article by a fitness expert who said if you could control your weight the minute you are three pounds over your right weight, you would never get fat. She said some people did not view three pounds as that much weight gain. If those who felt that way asked their butcher to wrap up three pounds of fat so they could hold it in their hand, they would quickly start losing those three pounds. I agree with her.

If we keep the fat down in our diets, we will also keep the fat off our bodies. I recommend the "blue jean test" for motivation. Keep your favorite jeans handy and slip them on from time to time to see if they fit nicely. If you can continue to slip into them over the years, you are keeping the fat content in your body under control. This will help ensure your good health.

Winning the Battle of the Bulge

Since God planned that we need food to survive, then we must drop the notion once and for all that food is a sin.

Who can judge if I have sinned if I eat ice cream? We must be careful to walk in love, offering concern, friendship, and prayer to the overweight person. You know what I say, "Let him who has never eaten an Oreo cast the first stone!"

Let's view obesity or being overweight as a problem that can be corrected with exercise and diet. We should not allow the standards of the media and the world to become the measuring stick by which we decide whether a person is weak or strong. Our souls and spirits cannot be gauged by worldly standards.

The struggle with weight is in most cases not a spiritual one in which the forces of heaven and hell are pulling at some poor soul. Most of the time the battle is physiological.

For example, studies in the early 1980s revealed the interesting action of enzymes that cause fat to be stored. These enzymes, while relatively inactive during a diet, inexplicably kick into overtime as soon as the diet ends. That's why a diet alone will peel the pounds off, as long as you stay on the diet. But you cannot stay on a severe, low-calorie diet forever and live long. Unless you've been exercising regularly, the pounds will pile back on when the diet ends.

What's the Secret?

When I was a young woman—prior to my exercising and eating sensibly years—I would have tried anything to remain a slim 98 pounds. As a matter of fact, I did. I tried starving, diuretics, and eating only one food at a time like apples. I can tell you that the principles in this book are right and they work.

At age forty-seven, I have finally learned the secret to sensible weight loss, and I want to pass it on to you. When 50 to 60 percent of your diet is made up of complex carbohydrates and the fat content is low, you enjoy a nice, healthy appetite, food satisfies you, and you do not binge eat.

I firmly believe binge eating is brought about by crazy dieting—mostly by not eating enough food. I am never starved, and I enjoy excellent health. I have lots of energy and I don't go to bed at night feeling as if my own stomach is going to eat me.

Don't Rush It

Too many women try to rush the weight loss process by using purging techniques such as vomiting, laxatives, diuretics, fasting, and extreme exercising. These methods destroy health and induce fatigue, muscles cramps, loss of endurance, headaches, bloating, edema, and heart disturbances, just to name a few. *Never before have so many gotten so sick trying to stay so thin!*

What is needed is a sensible, balanced low-fat diet and regular exercise. You should be able to feel good about your body. Regular daily exercise and a good eating program will do this for you.

You can't improve your eating habits overnight. Gradually change your diet, giving yourself time to learn to "like" what you are doing. If you like it, you will continue to do it. If two weeks of dieting yields no weight loss, you can slightly decrease your calorie intake and keep going. Don't call yourself a failure and quit just because you're not losing as fast as you want to or as fast as someone else.

If you are someone who needs to lose more than a few pounds, don't expect miracles in the weight-loss game. Shedding excess poundage requires commitment, discipline, and time. Focus on the positive, don't get discouraged if you hit a temporary stalemate, and treat yourself to non-food rewards for achieving short-term goals. If you believe in yourself and in what God can do through you, you will see change.

7

Getting the Best of Your Appetite

Crash diets and low-carbohydrate regimens can harm the dieter or cause him to actually gain more unwanted weight in the process. Laxatives, diuretics, and diet pills are obviously not the way to chemically induce weight loss. Resorting to artificial sweeteners, diet sodas, and other low-cal foods may sap you of calories and nutrients.

Even though there are no shortcuts to shedding excess poundage, a smart dieter understands the way his body works and takes advantage of that information. In this chapter we will discuss scheduling meals, the importance of breakfast, lunch, and dinner, and hunger satisfaction.

When Do You Eat?

Scientists are now suggesting that the time of day we eat may play a prominent role in weight gain. In one recent study, subjects were fed 2,000 calories per day for two weeks. During the first week, they ate all 2,000 calories at breakfast. During the second week, they ate all calories at supper.

During the week of breakfast eating, the subjects averaged *losing* 2.2 pounds. During the week of supper, two-thirds of the subjects *gained* weight and one-third lost insignificant amounts. Both weeks the diets were exactly the same. The only difference was the time of day when the food was eaten.

Scientists believe the weight loss was temperature related. The human body temperature is lowest at night and peaks during the day. Temperature is controlled by metabolism. When metabolism is up, your temperature is up and more calories are burned.

As a result of these and other studies, scientists feel that the calories we consume early in the day are more likely to be burned and those consumed in the evening are more likely to be stored as fat.

The old saying, "Eat breakfast like a king, lunch like a prince, and dinner like a pauper," holds true today. If you think about it, this is just the opposite to the American lifestyle in most homes.

Your Number One Meal of the Day

Too many Americans get the cart before the horse in their eating habits. For example, a doughnut and coffee for breakfast, a sandwich and salad for lunch, and a huge "meat and potatoes" supper is the average pattern. This is just the opposite of what our bodies need.

Breakfast should be your biggest meal. After going without food all night, your body is in dire need of complete nourishment to supply you with maximum energy and strength for the day. Eating a doughnut and coffee for breakfast is like trying to run a car on vinegar.

USDA studies have shown that a lifetime of regular breakfasts is associated with vigorous old age in men and women. Other studies show that breakfast eaters have a faster reaction time throughout the morning and less midday fatigue than those who start the day with just coffee.

Studies have shown that breakfast eaters also show a higher job performance than non-eaters. This becomes especially obvious in children. Children who do not get a good breakfast are more listless, show low problem-solving abilities, and are irritable. When you stop to think that they haven't eaten all night, their blood sugar is low, and their growing young bodies are in need of fuel, it's no wonder they have problems in school.

"But I'm Not Hungry at Breakfast"

If that's your complaint, stop eating at night. People who don't eat breakfast start feeling tired and dull around eleven o'clock in the morning. Brown bag a breakfast to work.

If you simply cannot stand to eat a large, hearty breakfast, try eating two small breakfasts during the morning. Yogurt and fresh fruit, for example, are a great way to start the day. Later eat a bran muffin. By furnishing your body with some badly-needed fuel, you will think more clearly and function better throughout the morning.

Testing has shown that even long-time breakfast skippers who began eating a morning meal started feeling like they had the wind at their backs. Their mornings became a breeze.

Won't I Gain Weight?

Going without food triggers the body's starvation mechanisms, making your metabolism slow down and hindering the use of stored fat for energy. Not eating in the morning can lead to a rise in blood cholesterol and wide gaps in blood sugar and insulin levels.

Skipping breakfast to help you lose weight is only a myth. A good breakfast can assist you in losing weight and in lengthening your life. A nutritious start each day can improve job performance and your sense of well being.

Skipping breakfast always backfires on dieters. Your early morning good intentions leave you so famished that later you will eat anything. Late evening meals cause you to store calories as fat. Calories eaten early are burned. You don't need a lot of calories at breakfast—200-500 will do.

What Is a Good Breakfast?

A good breakfast should contain about one-third of your daily protein needs. For the average adult, this would be equivalent to four tablespoons of peanut butter or two cups of milk.

To fulfill your *fruit requirements,* you need:

—a whole orange or one-half cup of orange juice;
—or one-half grapefruit;
—or one-half cup of strawberries;
—or one-fourth of a melon or cantaloupe.

Add some complex carbohydrates like whole grain bread or cereal or muffins made from bran or oats and some milk for calcium and you will have a healthy breakfast.

Breakfast is the best meal to eat vitamin C, calcium, and riboflavin. The body makes most use of them then.

What is a good breakfast?

1. A meal that provides steady energy throughout the morning.
2. A meal that keeps you alert and calm.
3. A meal low in fat and salt and not too high in calories that takes the edge off a lunchtime feeding frenzy.

Grains are the best way to start the day and are superior in many ways to the fast-food combos using eggs, sausage, ham, bacon, and cheese. Nutrition surveys say if you prefer cereal for breakfast, you probably have better-than-average dietary habits during the rest of the day. Cereal eaters consume less fat, less cholesterol, less salt, and fewer calories than those who start with different fare.

In a hurry? Try your regular cereal with some fruit and low-fat milk. Or try yogurt or cottage cheese with fruit, granola, raisins or all three. Even peanut butter on whole wheat bread is better than coffee and doughnuts.

Right foods at breakfast can mean energy, alertness, and hunger control far into the day. Ask a nutritionist what she eats for breakfast and the answer will be cereal—hot or cold with skim milk. It's fast, light, and right. Cereal meets all the requirements of a good breakfast.

Lunch: Your Second Most Important Meal

If you skip lunch, you will pay for it later in the afternoon. True, skipping your midday meal will prevent the usual dip in performance and drowsy feeling that is so common right after lunch. But later your energy will drop drastically.

A light but nutritionally balanced lunch will not dull your concentration and will allow you to keep your energy. Your midday meal should meet one-third of your daily protein needs. You will also need a good dose of complex carbohydrates.

Some people do their worst eating at lunch. They take whatever happens to be handy—greasy fries, a burger, or "fried anything." The best thing to do is pack your own lunch of soup or leftover supper from the night before, some celery, carrot sticks, and fruit. You might prefer a sandwich of leftover meat with lettuce or a salad and fruit with yogurt or cottage cheese.

Supper: Lean and Light

Supper or dinner should be the lightest and smallest meal of the day. Just about anything you eat for supper will end up being stored as fat unless you exercise after you eat. Unless you eat by five or six o'clock and remain active until at least nine or ten o'clock, supper should be light.

If you have the standard meal of a meat and two vegetables, keep the portions small. Have your smallest portion of protein at this time and fill in with starchy foods. If you do, you will sleep much better because carbohydrates stimulate a process that ends with the brain producing serotonin—the natural sleep inducer. Too much protein blocks the production of serotonin.

If you have a sweet tooth, go ahead and have a candy bar, a little ice cream, or cake perhaps once a week. (Only if you know you are not addicted to sugar.) Sometimes a few sweets from time to time will keep you from developing a wild craving and binging on a whole cake.

If you are addicted to sugar, stay away from those snacks entirely. Just one bite of something sweet can send a sugarholic on a sweets binge that will undo weeks of diet and exercise—not to mention the damage to one's self-esteem. I stay away from sweets altogether. Fresh fruit will usually curb a craving for sweets anyway. I always have fruit.

Do You Know When You're Full?

Hunger lets you know when it is time to get something to eat. If the biological mechanism that controls hunger malfunctions, you may not know if you have eaten enough. You may continue eating long after you are full. Controlling the feeling of hunger makes it much easier to stick to a sensible diet and lose weight.

The opposite of hunger is a feeling of being satisfied. The stomach plays the most important part in your feelings of hunger or being satisfied. Chemical and stretch receptors in the stomach signal the brain to stop eating when enough food has been consumed. These receptors are buried in the pits and folds of the mucous membrane that lines the stomach and small intestine.

As the stomach becomes full, it stretches and expands, activating the stretch and chemical receptors. When stimulated, these receptors trigger the secretion of hormones called peptides, which are released into the bloodstream where they flow to the brain.

These hormones signal the brain that you are full and that it's time to stop eating. Insulin, one of the peptide hormones, is believed to be the primary messenger that notifies the brain that the stomach is full.

Is It Soup Yet?

One way to induce satiety involves figuring out which foods fill you up. In some controlled studies, subjects were given a pre-load of some food before eating and were allowed to eat until they felt full. The best pre-load foods were soups. Tomato soup was found to be four times more effective than popular liquid diet meals or even cake. If you don't like tomato, chicken noodle soup is just as effective.

Soup is really an anti-appetizer—it cuts appetite rather than stimulates it. Soup has fewer calories than more dense foods and it takes longer to eat. The warmth of soup expands the volume of the stomach, and the salt increases thirst. Drinking water or tea will cut the appetite. With soup, the brain has time to register that you have eaten, and you consequently feel satisfied sooner and eat less.

If a meal starts with soup, fewer total calories will be consumed. Consuming soup with your midday meal helps reduce the calories eaten at lunch *and* at dinner! Studies also show that those who regularly eat soup are better able to maintain their weight losses than those who do not.

Learn What Fills You Up

Other research has shown that different forms of the same food can slow down calorie consumption. For example, you will probably eat less baked potato than french fries because it usually takes longer to eat a baked potato; less apple than applesauce; less orange than orange juice; and less green salad than potato salad.

High-fiber foods also contribute to feelings of satiety because they absorb water and expand in the stomach during the meal. This is why Chinese food is so satisfying. It's high-bulk, low-calorie, and salty.

No food can completely curb your appetite because appetite, to the greatest extent, is controlled by the mind. Learn what foods fill you up and which ones contain the most nutrients with the least amount of calories.

Hunger Satisfaction and Dieting

An Englishman once said, "The belly has no ears when hunger comes upon it." You might be dieting but when you are starved, you forget all about your promises and start eating like crazy.

You must feel satisfied after eating. What helps you feel satisfied? How do you keep the calories and fat intake down? Here are some suggestions.

1. Don't have too much variety. Too much food encourages overeating.
2. Your body knows when you have eaten fat. A little fat and a little sugar, when well-measured, can help you feel satisfied on fewer calories.
3. All food components help you feel satisfied— carbohydrates (both simple and complex), proteins, and fats.

Fat slows the exit of food from your stomach by tightening the pyloric valve, the stomach's outlet to the small intestine. When food lingers in your stomach a feeling of fullness promotes satiety.

Dairy products promote satiety. These contain shorter chain triglycerides that go quickly to the liver. In just a matter of minutes these fats get absorbed and turned into energy. The liver gets its nutrients from the intestines and sends electrical signals to the brain through nerves to let the body know it has consumed enough calories for now.

Curbing Your Appetite

We eat primarily for energy, so when our brains get feedback that we are getting plenty of energy, we feel satisfied. For best results, eat a small amount of fat early in the meal.

Carbohydrates play an important role in satiety. Fruits, whole grains, and vegetables will help you feel satisfied. Try a fruit dessert at the beginning of a meal. Pineapple, for example, is high in fructose. Since evidence suggests that the liver utilizes fructose quickly, it should play an important role in curbing appetite if eaten early in the meal.

Eating a sweet early in a meal gives a psychological satiety because we associate sweets with the end of the meal— with satisfaction. A fruit dessert provides bulk and fiber, which will also promote a feeling of fullness.

Studies show that high-carbohydrate dieters eat fewer calories than those who chomp on more calorie-rich foods. Fiber, vegetables, and whole grains are valuable assets to any weight loss program.

Outsmarting Your Appetite

If you want to be a smart and sensible dieter, don't skip breakfast. The calories you hope to save will only return to haunt you later in the day. Three nutritionally sound meals are a must, but eat your heartiest meal in the morning. Your metabolism will have the rest of the day to burn off those calories.

You don't have to be controlled by food cravings and hunger pangs. Try ignoring the urge to snack between meals— within minutes the hunger pangs often disappear. A glass of water may be all that you need until your next meal.

Learn to outsmart your appetite by starting out with soups, low-calorie fiber foods, or fruit that will fill you up and satisfy your hunger. For the knowledgeable dieter who understands how her body works, dieting doesn't have to be torture.

8

The Key to Lasting Weight Loss

Would you believe me if I told you that you could eat less meat and more starches like potatoes, bread, rice, and pasta without fear of gaining weight? Would you believe that you can feel full and satisfied after a meal and still be able to lose weight?

Would you like to kiss diet pills, powders, and schemes goodbye forever? Would you like to be slim and healthy without giving up some of your favorite foods? Sound too good to be true? Read on to see how it's done.

A high-carbohydrate, high-fiber, low-fat diet is the answer. Our bodies were designed to thrive on this type of diet. In parts of the world where people live the longest, they generally eat such a diet.

In fact, Americans have only recently strayed from a high-fiber, high-carbohydrate diet. Until this century, Americans existed on a plant-based diet of grains, beans, peas, nuts, potatoes, vegetables, and fruits. Now our dietary emphasis is placed on meat, fish, poultry, eggs, and dairy products. This is more costly calorie-wise, health-wise, and money-wise.

You may ask, "What do you mean? Don't Americans live longer now than ever before?" Yes, but not that much longer. Since the turn of the century, the life expectancy of males has increased approximately four years and that of females approximately seven years. Many of those who survive to age seventy are plagued with diet and lifestyle-related illnesses.

A 1982 report of the National Research Council of the National Academy of Sciences stated that 50 percent of the ten leading causes of death are directly related to lifestyle. The present way of eating in America increases the risk of heart disease, cancer, high blood pressure, stroke, diabetes, osteoporosis, and obesity.

Serving meat with every meal almost seems to be a social rule. This sign of hospitality may be a dangerous social habit. We are literally eating ourselves to death. The way out of this dilemma is to switch the emphasis from meats and fats to carbohydrates.

What Are Carbohydrates?

Carbohydrates are the chief source of energy for all body functions and muscular exertions. They are also a necessary part of the digestion and assimilation of other foods. They provide immediate energy so the body can save protein for the building and repairing of tissues. They help regulate protein and fat metabolism.

Carbohydrates come in three forms: sugars, starches, and cellulose. All sugars and starches are converted by the digestive juices to simple sugar called glucose or "blood sugar."

Simple sugars such as those found in honey and fruit are easily digested. Some are used for immediate energy to support the basic functions of breathing, heartbeat, and cell activity.

Some are used as fuel for tissues of the brain, nervous system, and muscles. A small amount is converted to glycogen and stored in the liver and muscles. The excess is converted to fat and stored throughout the body as a reserve source of energy. An individual begins to lose weight when his fat reserves are reconverted to glucose and used for body fuel.

Starches require a great deal more processing in order to be broken down into simple sugars (or glucose) for digestion. Cellulose, found in the skins of fruits and vegetables, is for the most part indigestible by humans and contributes little in the way of energy. Cellulose does, however, provide bulk and fiber that is necessary for proper action of the intestines and bowels.

Eating sweet carbohydrate snacks provides the body with instant energy. After bringing on a sudden rise in the blood sugar level, however, simple carbohydrates cause the blood sugar to drop again rapidly. This results in a craving for more sweets and symptoms of fatigue, dizziness, nervousness, and headache. Craving sugar can cause an individual to eat more and to fall into a dangerous pattern of craving, snacking, low blood sugar, and weight gain.

Complex Carbohydrates

When properly prepared, complex carbohydrates are the only foods that you can eat in large proportion and not harm your health. As much as 80 percent of your diet can safely come from this food group.

Complex carbohydrates speed up the body's metabolism and are not likely to be stored as fat. Greater energy is required to digest and process carbohydrates than fats. In fact, a diet high in complex carbohydrates seems to stimulate the metabolism in much the same way as exercise and helps one maintain high energy at a lower body weight.

The energy found in carbohydrates such as pasta is stored in small amounts in the muscles and liver, and in normal cases, is almost never turned into fat. If you have to binge,

binge on complex carbohydrates. The body must burn 23 calories to turn 100 calories of carbohydrates into fat. That's good news!

Do Carbohydrates Convert To Fat?

Long ago an Iowa pig farmer noticed a change in his livestock when he stopped feeding them scraps containing animal by-products and saturated fats. When he began feeding them corn oil and soy products, the consistency of the swines' body fat became softer. This suggested to scientists that body fat has similar characteristics to the fat we eat—either saturated or unsaturated. This discovery led some investigators to go one step further.

Researchers surmised the fat we store in our bodies must be coming from the fat in our diets. If dietary fat is deposited in our fat cells, what happens to the carbohydrates? Studies were done to see if we ever convert carbohydrates into fat.

Humans and animals make very small amounts of body fat from the carbohydrates they eat. A significant conversion of carbohydrates into body fat occurs only under conditions where astronomical amounts of carbohydrates and no fat at all are eaten.

For instance, if you were to sit down and eat 2,000 calories of carbohydrates in one meal—just carbohydrates—only 9 grams would end up as body fat. The fat in your body comes mainly from the fat you eat—not from the carbohydrates you eat.

Our bodies are just not equipped to store carbohydrates. Excess carbohydrates are turned into glycogen. We can only store about one-half to one pound of glycogen in the muscles and liver. Our bodies know they have been fed when we eat carbohydrates because our metabolism begins to whir. That signal is given by insulin, which is triggered by the ingestion of carbohydrates.

If you eat spaghetti or potatoes, your body knows you have eaten. Metabolically speaking, eating carbohydrates stimulates the nervous system, slightly increases the heart rate, and speeds up all body processes.

Carbohydrates Burn More Calories

Carbohydrates increase the thermic effect or calorie-burning abilities of food. Your temperature rises slightly when you eat. This is why, when you walk into a restaurant you may feel cool, but you feel much warmer after your meal. Producing this heat costs extra energy, which results in burning more calories. Both proteins and carbohydrates increase body temperature, but fats do not.

You can eat fats all day and never feel quite satisfied because your body has not received a clear message that it has eaten. Fats can't deliver a message that only insulin-inducing carbohydrates were meant to send.

Don't get the impression, however, that you can lose weight indefinitely on a low-fat, high-carbohydrate diet. Eventually you will reach a new, lower set weight. If you stick to the low-fat regimen and regular exercise, you can maintain your set weight indefinitely.

Can I Eat Bread?

Yes, you can! In the past, when a person wanted to diet, the first foods cut from the diet were bread, rice, potatoes, and pasta. Instead, they would try to live on meat, salad, cottage cheese, vegetables, and fruits. Before long, they would begin to feel depressed, tired, and even ill. Sometimes sleep eluded these frustrated dieters. What was happening?

The body was saying, "Hey, I have to have some carbohydrates in here!" As a result of setting up defense mechanisms against starvation, the brain had stopped manufacturing serotonin, a carbohydrate-induced hormone that helps induce sleep and calmness.

When your body needs a nutrient in order to survive, it will crave that nutrient. A dieter begins to crave carbohydrates so badly that at the first smell of cake or pizza, his resolve and determination is drowned in a outcry from the body of, "Yes! Yes! That's what I've been needing!"

The dieter gives in to his carbohydrate-depleted body and eats and eats and eats. Since the brain has prepared the body for starvation, the metabolism is slowed. The calories that would normally burn off just pile back on—as fat.

Including starches in your diet can actually help you control your weight because it keeps the body from craving and starving. If you fill up on starches, you feel full and satisfied without having to eat a lot of meat or sweets.

Good examples of breads you can eat are whole wheat, rye, and pita. I prefer pita bread, which can be bought from the deli section of most food stores. Pita bread has almost no fat.

Eat the Bun, Leave the Hamburger

The dieter who eats the hamburger and leaves the bun thinks he is doing the right thing. But he would be better off to eat the bun and leave the hamburger! Back in the 1950s studies showed that eating a high-protein meal raised the body's heat production and increased metabolic activity. No one bothered to mention that this increase in metabolism lasted only a few minutes, so a wave of high-protein diets ensued that are still prevalent today.

Today, nutritionists know that carbohydrates are most helpful in controlling weight and boosting metabolism around the clock. Calorie for calorie, carbohydrates lead to less fat storage than proteins. That's why a meal of fresh fruits, vegetables, and whole-grain breads or cereals is superior to a hamburger patty and cottage cheese.

You might say, "Well, when I eat bread, potatoes, rice, and spaghetti, I pile on the pounds." Starches themselves aren't responsible for weight gain, but what we put on them can make good diet foods quite fattening. Greasy spaghetti sauce over noodles, butter or sour cream on baked potatoes, and rich gravy on rice make you fat. But starches eaten with low-fat accompaniments remain low in fat.

Starch—A Good Diet Food

A survey by the Wheat Industry Council asked if people thought they should avoid starch when on a diet. Half of those surveyed thought they should. Surprised by those results?

If you had that same preconceived idea, I hope you are beginning to think differently now. I have listed below several reasons why starch is a good diet food.

1. The body must break down complex carbohydrates into glucose before it can use it for energy. This breaking down process burns 25 percent of the calories. Fat, on the other hand, burns only 3 percent. This means if you eat 100 calories of fat, 97 of them will be stored as fat.

2. Complex carbohydrates make a great diet food because they are stored in the liver and muscles as energy and cannot be stored as body fat.

3. Pound for pound or gram for gram, complex carbohydrates contain 44 percent fewer calories than fats.

4. Complex carbohydrates are nutritionally dense. They pack a lot of nutrients in a small caloric package. They are full of vitamins and minerals that enable the body to get the most nutrition for its calories.

5. Carbohydrates are satisfying. They stimulate secretion of insulin, which tells the body you are full. Fat does not do this. This is why you can eat nuts until you are stuffed and still not feel full. An apple provides a sense of being satisfied because it stimulates the production of insulin.

6. Complex carbohydrates are high in fiber. Fiber contains no available calories since it is indigestible material, but it does provide bulk to give a sense of fullness.

What Is Fiber?

Dietary fiber is the indigestible cell wall of plants. There are five kinds of fiber that provide important functions for the body.

Cellulose and hemicellulose are the fibers in bran, the outer husk of cereal grains. They are not soluble in water but they do absorb water like a sponge, increasing the water content of waste material as it moves through the intestines. This type of fiber speeds elimination.

Pectin is water soluble and is found in apples, pears, plums, figs, prunes, citrus fruits, bananas, and in some vegetables such as cabbage and cauliflower. Pectin slows the absorption of carbohydrates and combines with bile acids to prevent the absorption of cholesterol.

Lignin, found in mature vegetables and cereal grains, reduces the digestibility of all other fibers and helps keep cholesterol levels down.

Gum, which is found in oatmeal, helps control cholesterol.

Experts believe the typical American diet provides only half the fiber we need. While it is entirely possible to overdo with fiber, nutritionists believe it should be a part of every meal.

Here are some good sources of fiber:

Fruits—apricots, dates, raspberries, blackberries, strawberries, citrus fruits, apples, pears, plums, prunes, raisins, cherries, and bananas.

Vegetables—Dried peas, dried beans and other legumes, lima beans, broccoli, potatoes, green beans, turnip greens, spinach, brussels sprouts, corn, green peas.

Grains—Whole wheat and other whole-grain cereals and breads, and oatmeal.

Fiber is the part of carbohydrates that helps give you that satisfied, filled-up feeling without the calories. We were not meant to eat processed foods such as corn flakes. Our bodies function best on whole grains. Processed foods keep us hungry and don't satisfy the appetite until we have taken in excessive amounts of them.

Studies show that the average American diet requires 3,000 calories for appetite satisfaction. When fed a low-fat, high-fiber diet, the same individual is satisfied with only 1,500 calories.

Besides being bulky, fiber takes longer to consume. Both the bulk and the added chewing time help your brain give the signal of satisfaction. When including fiber in your diet, you will find you eat less calories and less food altogether.

Digesting fiber enables the body to feel full longer because it takes the stomach and small intestines longer to deal with it. Since fiber remains in the stomach longer than most food, it absorbs water. Then when it finally reaches the large intestine, it allows for easy, healthy bowel action. All this at no cost—no fat—no pounds. This is why fiber is so important in the prevention of colon diseases and cancer.

A pound of food stretches the stomach, distends the abdomen, and signals the brain that enough food has been ingested. A pound of oranges will stretch the stomach at a cost of only 200 calories. A pound of chocolate creams will do the same, but at ten times the calorie cost. A low-fat, high-fiber diet can't be beat for controlling weight and preventing disease.

Benefits of Fiber

Research has shown that a high-bulk diet is a great weapon against obesity. The *type* of food a person selects may make him obese, not necessarily the *amount* of food consumed.

A high-fiber diet pushes food through the body at a faster rate. This reduces calorie absorption and picks up fat on the way, decreasing the amount of fat absorbed by the body during digestion. Fiber helps keep insulin levels steady, which aids in less fat storage also. Fiber is believed to be beneficial in lowering levels of cholesterol in the blood. Doctors are prescribing a high-fiber, high-carbohydrate diet more and more for their diabetic and ulcer patients.

Since a high-carbohydrate diet promotes storage of muscle fuel, professional athletes who once ate lots of red meat for energy now follow the high-carbohydrate routine. Coaches now encourage spaghetti dinners for energy rather than steaks.

The only drawback to this diet is the excess gas it may produce in the bowels. At first you may experience a problem with this, but in most cases the gas will gradually subside over a period of a few weeks. I suggest you don't jump right into a high-fiber, high-complex carbohydrate diet but rather gradually add them to your diet.

Part Three
Eating and Exercising Right

9

The Diet Busters

Watch any old Western movie, and the plots are pretty similar. The bad guys saunter into town, cause trouble, and are pursued by the good guys. The movie always climaxes in a showdown that leaves the good guys standing. You can always spot the good guys because they're the clean-shaven fellows in the white hats.

Nutritionally speaking, knowing the good guys from the bad guys is not always that easy. Too often we're unaware of fat content in our favorite foods. The result? We're siding with the bad guys who are wrecking our diets and health.

Jane Brody, in her *Good Food Book,* lists the ten worst foods to eat, according to fat content and nutritional value. Some of your favorite foods may be on this list.

The Worst Foods List

1. *Soda pop*—Nutritionally, all carbonated soft drinks score a big zero. Sugar sweetened or artificially sweetened beverages are no exception. If you need a sweet drink, try fruit juice.

2. *French fries*—The wonderful potato becomes a dead weight of 200 empty calories when fried. In fast food restaurants, french fries are usually cooked in beef tallow and dowsed in salt.

3. *Potato chips*—Jane Brody says you might as well eat butter. Potato chips contain huge amounts of fat and salt.

4. *Bacon*—Ninety-five percent of the calories in bacon come from fat, thereby disqualifying it as a meat. Bacon also contains unwanted salt and nitrates.

5. *Pasta salads*—Pasta is great until you drown it in fatty sauces.

6. *Fast-food burgers*—Whoppers and Big Macs can easily pack 600 calories and half of them are fat. Plain burgers are not so bad, but when you throw in the dressing, cheese, and an extra beef patty, the fat content skyrockets.

7. *Granola bars*—Granola is high-fat and high-sugar. Granola bars are high-calorie cookies. You might as well eat a Milky Way when you bite into a granola bar.

8. *Sugar-sweetened cereals*—Read the labels on the cereal boxes. Some are no better than eating candy with milk on it.

9. *Doughnuts*—Worse than no breakfast at all, says Jane. Those fried and coated pastries contain no nutritive value, just sugar and fat. Eating doughnuts are a good way to have a bad morning.

10. *Cheese*—Many people have replaced meat with cheese, thinking they have reduced their cholesterol intake. But cheese has the same amount of fat and cholesterol as red meat and far more salt. Cream cheese is one of the worst cheeses you can eat. The best cheeses are low-fat cottage, part-skim mozzarella, skim milk ricotta, and feta cheese.

Sugar: One of the Bad Guys

Sugar abuse is probably the most underrated health threat today. For a substance that has little or no nutritional value, sugar plays far too large a role in the average American diet.

Did you know that the average American eats over two pounds of sugar a day—just from processed foods to which sugar has been added—foods like ketchup which is 63 percent sugar and cranberry sauce which is 96 percent sugar? Did you know a fondness for sweets is "inborn"—that babies a day old will prefer sweet water to plain?

One-fifth to one-fourth of the calories we take in daily come from sugar-prepared foods. These are empty, useless calories.

One would think that with all the bad publicity sugar gets, it would be the cause of all kinds of cancers and illnesses. But the only disease with which sugar alone has a proven link is tooth decay. Surprised?

While sugar is not the direct cause of any diseases other than tooth decay, it does increase the damaging effects of such diseases as diabetes. Sugar keeps bad company with fat, and fat causes all kinds of illnesses.

Tests have also proven that sugar can adversely affect a person's performance levels. For example, runners were given a sugared drink in one study and asked to ride a stationary bike to exhaustion. Three days later they were given a sugar-free drink and asked to ride to exhaustion. They were able to ride the bike 25 percent longer with a sugar-free drink.

Sugar also seems to irritate the bowels. Up to 30 percent of those who suffer from bowel irritations do so because of a high-sugar diet. By the way, did you know that 12 ounces of Pepsi contains ten teaspoons of sugar? Just some food for thought.

Sugar Addiction

Our bodies do not need sugar at all, yet we continue to pour an estimated 120 pounds of it into us each year. Of all the forms in which we can eat sugar—brown sugar, honey, raw sugar, white sugar—only molasses can boast of having any nutrients. Most sweet foods are high in fat, so in order for a body to metabolize sugar, it must use up valuable vitamins and minerals. Sugar is not only useless, it is, indirectly, harmful.

Sugar does not satisfy hunger, and those who eat a high-sugar diet tend to overeat in an effort to feel satisfied. Some people are convinced they need the "high" or quick energy that only sugar can give them. This short-lived high usually leaves the person feeling worse once it fades. Most people usually feel irritable and weak within one hour of having indulged heavily in sweets.

Can a person really be addicted to sugar? If you can't stop with one candy bar but instead eat three or even six, then you know the answer to that question. An addiction to sugar can be just as strong as an addiction to alcohol.

Sugar does make you feel good temporarily. Not long after swallowing candy you feel a nice euphoria and a burst of energy. When that quickly wears off, it's time for more candy and more pounds.

Food addiction works the same as drug addiction. The addict shoots up, feels great, starts feeling bad, and shoots up again. Sugar addiction is no different. Of course, not everyone who eats sugar is addicted to it. When you can't get along without it for more than a few hours, though, you are in trouble.

What Causes Addiction?

One doctor who works with drug addicts, alcoholics, and food addicts has said that their symptoms are so similar it is hard to tell who is addicted to what.

Endorphins, a hormone that acts on the brain and nerves to lessen pain and elevate mood, is connected to all addictions. Drugs, alcohol, and nicotine act as substitutes for endorphins, and like food abuse, can upset the endorphin balance. Research shows that sugar apparently depresses endorphins. As your body metabolizes sugar, the blood sugar falls. When the short high disappears, your body craves sugar to recapture the euphoric feelings.

Endorphin sites are found in the part of the brain that affects hunger, thirst, and emotions. But, if drugs, alcohol, or nicotine are locked into your receptor sites in your brain, they will block out your natural endorphin high. Exercise produces a natural high. Substance and food abuse block out this natural endorphin high.

Sugar depresses endorphins and is absolutely addictive. Someone may say, "My problem is sweets; a candy bar every day is no big deal." Science tells us it is a big deal because you are becoming addicted.

Such addictions often spring from unfulfilled emotional needs and general unhappiness. The best answer is to find happiness and emotional stability in constructive outlets such as taking up a new hobby, receiving counseling, reading Scripture, and praying. Your sense of well-being should not hinge on anything as powerless and meaningless as a chemical or a food.

Kicking The Habit

Realize that you can make a difference in your feelings without food or chemicals. Develop good habits of exercise and eating. Drink eight to twelve glasses of water a day. The natural high from exercise is a lift that you can treat yourself to every day without harm. Exercise reduces stress and allows your mind and body to work efficiently. If you are fighting a food addiction, you will need to exercise daily. Two or three times a week won't do it.

When you get the craving for sweets, take a brisk, thirty-minute walk. If you can't walk, drink water. Once an addict, always an addict. You may have to stay away from sugar entirely, or you will rekindle the habit. After seven to ten days without sugar, the addiction is temporarily broken and the withdrawal ended.

Never think that artificial sweeteners are a substitute for sugar. They will not help you break your addiction; they will only serve to increase your craving.

One study has raised the possibility that some people may have a biochemical need for carbohydrates, specifically sugars and starches, that no amount of willpower or dieting can curb.

Researchers devised a diet with the sweets craver in mind. They proposed that a 1,100-calorie daily diet can harbor 200 calories of carbohydrates that can come from a candy bar, dried raisins, one ounce of potato chips, or a brownie or muffin. These snacks must be eaten alone—not as dessert— and must be eaten slowly to allow the brain time to register their presence and thus decrease the chance of overeating them. This works for some people.

Gradually Phasing Sugar Out

If you feel the desire to have sweets and you know you are not addicted to them, it is okay to occasionally indulge. But there is one word of caution. Be sure you have offset the negative effects of sweets by following a high-fiber, high-complex carbohydrate, low-fat diet. A sweet every so often may keep you from feeling deprived and overindulging at a weak moment.

You can re-train your taste buds to prefer less sugary foods and to even dislike things that are too sweet. Don't get into trouble by over-sweetening. You can enjoy many of the same desserts you always have but with half the sugar. In most recipes you can easily cut the amount of sugar by one-third to one-half without changing the taste or texture significantly.

Start gradually. First, get away from desserts with sugary frostings. Instead try more fruit tarts or coffee cakes. Before you know it, you will find yourself repulsed by any heavy, sugary taste.

Second, forget the myth that you need sugar for high energy. A high energy level can be achieved with a high-carbohydrate, low-fat diet and regular exercise. If you want to cut back on sweets, follow these tips and you will experience success.

1. For dessert or snacks, choose fruit. Fresh is best. Avoid canned fruits in heavy, sweet syrups.

2. Drink unsweetened juices. If you like the soda taste, mix your own soda by adding one-half glass of club soda to one-half glass of your favorite juice.

3. Rather than buying ready-made desserts, try to make your own and use one-third to one-half less sugar than the recipe calls for.

4. Use plain yogurt and sweeten it with fresh fruit or juices.

5. Choose unsweetened cereals and sweeten them with fruit or raisins.

The Nicotine-Sugar Connection

Researchers say they have found a direct link between nicotine and sugar. In studies on rats and humans nicotine intake reduced the craving for sweet foods; without nicotine the same subjects experienced an increased desire for sweets.

Although all the answers are not yet in, studies indicate that the reason for this link may be due to the fact that nicotine affects the level of glucose in the body, which in turn would alter the craving for sweets.

If you don't want to quit smoking for fear of gaining weight, perhaps you could throw out all sweets first and then the cigarettes.

Artificial Sweeteners

One question I am often asked is, "Do artificial sweeteners help you lose weight?" I personally do not believe they do, and there is plenty of research that indicates I am right.

For example, the American Cancer Society and a British research team found that people who consumed sugar substitutes instead of the real thing still put on pounds. Using diet aids will not automatically make you lose weight.

Saving a few calories with a diet soda often lulls a dieter into a false sense of security. Thinking he has "saved" some calories, a dieter is more tempted to indulge in an occasional fattening ice cream sundae. I've seen people have a diet soda with a piece of pie or cake. Why bother? Why not just go ahead and have sugar in the drink as well?

Dieters who drink water as their main source of liquids fare much better in the weight loss game than those who guzzle diet sodas. Diet sodas tend to leave a sweet taste in the mouth and prepare the body for the digestion of a lot of calories. This is called "residual hunger." When those expected calories never arrive, the body sends out hunger signals that cause the dieter to crave food—especially high-calorie junk food.

Artificial sweeteners do nothing to curb a craving for sweets. In my opinion, diet sodas are just as harmful as sugared sodas—neither provide the body with anything it needs.

Satisfaction or Frustration?

The difference between a successful diet and one that fails is whether or not the dieter was able to feel satisfied after eating. If a dieter still feels hungry after he eats, sooner or later he is going to give in and satisfy that hunger.

A dieter certainly does not need anything that will increase his sense of hunger. Water satisfies and can even serve as an appetite suppressant. The sense of being full helps a dieter stick with his diet.

Results of tests now tell us that we eat by "weight" of the food not by the actual intake of calories. Foods like fruits, vegetables, whole grains, skim milk, and water work well for the dieter. The weight of the food in their stomach makes them feel satisfied and keeps down the cravings for fat, sugary foods.

If you are in a hurry and you must choose something quick, choose a frozen diet "something" rather than a frozen rich and gooey "something." Prepared diet foods that save calories do have their place.

Not all foods that call themselves "diet," however, are low in calories. For example, sugar-free does not necessarily mean lower in calories. There are artificial sweeteners on the market that contain just as many calories as sugar. Make sure you read all the labels carefully before eating.

Drawbacks to Artificial Sweeteners

Research has indicated that artificial sweeteners not only increase the craving for sweets but can actually drive up your body's set point—the weight your body maintains when you are doing nothing to lose.

Not only do artificial sweeteners not help in weight loss, they seem to encourage weight gain. Some of the people I've met with the worst weight problems were heavy users of artificial sweeteners. Some of the most successful weight losers did not use artificial sweeteners at all.

The most obvious reason not to use artificial sweeteners is because of the numerous studies that have indicated that saccharin, in particular, can cause cancer. Not enough work has been done to determine the effects of artificial sweeteners on humans. In light of the information available, why take a chance and use them at all?

Even sweeteners such as Equal and NutraSweet have been known to cause reactions as varied as depression, headaches, irritability, dizziness, and seizures.

Fructose, or the natural sugar present in fruit, is now being produced commercially for use as an artificial sweetener.

Natural and artificial fructose seem to be identical in chemical make-up, but the consumption of great amounts of artificial fructose has caused side effects such as bloating, diarrhea, and stomach pain. Nature never intended for the body to consume large amounts of fructose.

What About Imitation Foods?

More and more artificial foods are being made available to the public now, not just in the form of sweeteners. These substitutes—such as Tang, Coffeemate, breakfast sausages, bacon, and butter—resemble the real thing and even taste like it. But are they harmful?

Nutritionists say, "It depends." It depends on who you are and what you want to be health-wise. Fake foods are often lower in fat, calories, and cholesterol than their real counterparts. They can even be cheaper. For example, fake eggs are usually cheaper and go further than real eggs. But these fake foods are usually high in sodium and full of preservatives, artificial flavors, and colors. Worst of all, they usually lack important nutrients.

If people desperately need to omit fat, sugar, and cholesterol from their diets, imitation foods are useful. Not all are lacking in nutrients; some are vitamin fortified. But the real danger comes from not being able to duplicate nature completely. All elements in natural foods have yet to be identified. It is impossible, therefore, to completely duplicate any food.

Nutritionists recommend you not eat more than 20 to 25 percent of your diet in these low-value foods. To eat more than that would put you at risk of becoming deficient in valuable trace minerals and vitamins.

For example, imitation milk provides one-third to one-half the calcium of real milk, half the protein, twice the sodium, and significantly more sugar. It contains more saturated fat than real milk and sixteen times more fat than non-fat dry milk. Most nutritionists agree that sticking with the real thing is better when it comes to food. With care in preparation and serving, you can make natural foods work for you and your needs.

─── 10 ───
Potatoes and Pasta

If you knew you were going to be stranded on a desert island, what foods would you take with you? Jane Brody in her *Good Food Book* lists the ten best foods you can eat to stay healthy and trim. You may be surprised to find out what they are.

1. *Broccoli and carrots*—These vegetables are high in fiber and contain natural cancer-preventative agents. Cooked carrots are more easily absorbed by the body than raw.
2. *Oats*—This grain, being rich in protein and fiber, helps to reduce cholesterol and normalize blood sugar. Instant oatmeal is not as effective as cooked oatmeal because of added salt and sugar.
3. *Cabbage*—This family of vegetables, including cauliflower, brussels sprouts, and kale, reduces the risk of colon cancer.
4. *Potatoes*—Provide vitamin C, protein, iron, riboflavin, thiamine, niacin, phosphorus, and magnesium. Don't cook potatoes in fat or add sour cream or butter. Just put cooked vegetables on the potato and sprinkle on some low-fat cheese.

5. *Yogurt and skim milk*—These dairy products provide protein and calcium.

6. *Pasta*—Not a fattening food unless loaded down with cheeses and fatty sauces. Provides protein, vitamins, and minerals.

7. *Fish*—Excellent food. Eat it broiled without butter.

8. *Bread and whole grains*—No wonder bread is called the staff of life. These necessary foods should be part of every meal.

9. *Fresh fruit*—Fruits are a low-fat, natural dessert that will satisfy your taste for sweets and fill you up. They're loaded with fiber, vitamins, and minerals.

10. *Popcorn*—This light snack is great if unbuttered and unsalted. Popcorn has lots of fiber and only 23 calories per cup. Season it with herbs, parmesan cheese, or black pepper.

The Nutritious Potato

During the 1950s and 1960s potatoes were given an unfair reputation of being a "poor man's food"—something to fill an empty stomach but having no real nutritional value and no class.

How wrong! A medium-sized potato that is baked, boiled or steamed contains approximately 100 calories. That's low enough to suit the most discriminating nutritionist. Potatoes become fattening only when fried or smothered in butter, sour cream or sauces. Add some low-fat dairy products like yogurt or low-fat cheese along with greens to a potato, and you have a highly nutritious meal with few calories.

The skin of the potato is its most nutritious part. The outer layer of the potato contains nutrients like iron, magnesium, copper, niacin and vitamins C, B-1, and B-6. But the potato's flesh is also quite nutritious. If you want to know what to do with a potato, eat the whole thing.

Potatoes are low in sodium and contain almost 20 percent of your daily potassium needs, making them useful in preventing and treating high blood pressure. If that doesn't sell you—the protein found in potatoes is comparable to that found in beef.

When preparing potatoes, avoid frying them altogether. A serving of french fries, for example, contains the fat equivalent of two tablespoons of butter. Likewise, potato chips are disastrously fattening because of the oil and salt added to them.

Fix your own potatoes. You can control the fat and salt content by using skim milk, diet margarine, and little salt in preparation. Season potatoes with pepper, herbs, lemon juice or a low-calorie cheese instead of salt.

"I Owe it All to Spaghetti"

The beautiful actress Sophia Loren has been quoted as saying, "Everything you see, I owe to spaghetti." Pasta is leaving behind its reputation of being a fattening food and is fast becoming a favorite of champions, executives, housewives, and everyone who wants to eat well and stay fit. Pasta has what it takes to keep us lean and energetic.

A complex carbohydrate, pasta is low in calories and nearly fat-free—only 210 calories per cooked cup. Pasta is perfect for dieters who want to diet the healthy way. What few calories pasta does have are loaded with vitamins such as niacin, thiamin, and riboflavin with some protein and iron. Pasta has very little salt.

What is so great about pasta is the way it cooks up. Research has shown that pasta retains most of its mineral content after being cooked. Two cups give you the following percentages of the Recommended Dietary Allowance for six minerals:

    manganese—31 percent.
    iron—24 percent.

phosphorus—16 percent.
copper—16 percent.
magnesium—12 percent.
zinc—9 percent.

Pasta fills you up without your having to overeat. One cup of spaghetti, for example, has approximately 200 calories, less than half the calories of a steak of comparable weight. Spaghetti with a low-fat sauce, a salad, and fruit for dessert will satisfy you and taste good at the same time. You can fill up on pasta without feeling guilty. It is a slowly-digested food that takes the guilt out of eating until you are full. Just don't ruin pasta's good qualities by piling rich, fattening sauces on it.

What About Pasta Salads?

Hidden fat may be lurking in your pasta salad. A recent study revealed that a serving of pasta salad can have as much fat as almost three cups of ice cream. Twenty-four salads from supermarkets, fast-food restaurants, and the at-home package mixes were tested. The big losers were those with creamy Italian dressing that contained up to 9 teaspoons of fat in a 3/4 cup serving. Read the fat content on the box mixes to see how much fat they contain.

Why are some pasta salads so much more fattening than others? They are made with regular mayonnaise instead of oil. Ounce for ounce, oil has more fat than mayonnaise, but it takes less oil to coat the noodles.

Manufacturers of these pasta mixes have rested on the image of pasta salad being a healthy food and have failed to keep the fat content down. The same study has also found that salads vary widely in nutritional value. Some contain healthy doses of broccoli, carrots, and green peas, which are high in vitamins A and C. Others, however, are high in sodium and preservatives.

When looking for the benefits of pasta salad without the drawbacks, pay attention to ingredients. Better yet, boil some water, cook the pasta, chop up vegetables, and make your own.

A Nutrient Gold Mine

Beans have gained a new respectability of late and are no longer considered "poor man's fare." As people become more nutrition-conscious, they realize that beans are a nutrient gold mine.

Beans provide many times more protein and a fraction of the fats and cholesterol of meat. Beans go with a lot of other foods and can be easily and tastily added to salads and casseroles. Beans have no cholesterol, actually *lower* existing cholesterol levels, control diabetes, and act as a natural laxative.

Some people avoid beans because they take so long to cook and because they cause intestinal gas. Once you realize what beans can do for you, I don't think you'll mind the preparation time. There are also proven ways to diminish the gaseous discomforts associated with beans.

The more beans you eat, the less bloating and discomfort they cause. Your body adjusts to them. Because beans affect each person differently, don't assume you can't enjoy them just because someone else cannot.

More For Your Money

Beans are definitely the most healthful and least expensive way to meet your protein needs. Beans (all legumes including peas, soybeans, peanuts, and lentils) are also rich in B vitamins and iron. To get the most iron out of beans, eat them with vitamin C-rich foods such as broccoli, tomatoes, and citrus fruits. Other good things in beans include calcium and phosphorus.

Beans boast a high nutritive value combined with low fat and low sodium content. The minimal fat in beans is polyunsaturated and harmless. A cup of cooked beans is only 4 percent fat; most red meats contain 60 percent fat.

Beans are also high in fiber—so high that only cereal bran exceeds them. The bean is a complete food containing starches, complex sugars, and dietary fiber. The starches in beans help control blood sugar. In fact, studies have shown that diabetics can actually reduce their need for insulin by including large amounts of legumes in their diets.

Complex carbohydrates like beans are digested slowly, causing increased burning of calories during digestion while giving the brain time to register the news to the body that it has eaten and is full.

What About Protein?

Protein is very important in our diets for the maintenance of good health and vitality and is of primary importance in the growth and development of all body tissues. Protein is the major source of building material for muscles, blood, skin, hair, nails, and internal organs, including the heart and brain.

Protein is needed for the formation of hormones that control a variety of body functions. Protein helps prevent the blood and tissues from becoming either too acidic or too alkaline and helps regulate the body's water balance. Enzymes, substances necessary for basic life functions, and antibodies, which help fight foreign substances in the body, are also formed from protein.

As well as being the major source of building material for the body, protein may be used as a source of heat and energy, providing four calories per gram of protein. This energy function is diminished, however, when sufficient fats and carbohydrates are present in the diet. Excess protein that is not used for building tissue or energy can be converted by the liver and stored as fat in the body tissues.

Sources of Protein

Soybeans are perfect protein. They produce more protein per acre than any other plant or animal. Soybeans could easily supply the total protein needs of our entire nation at less the cost and land required for animals.

Soy protein can also bring about a reduction in blood cholesterol levels because the fat in soybeans is different from that found in meat and animal products. It is highly unsaturated. The fat in meat and cheeses is saturated and raises blood cholesterol.

Nuts and seeds are costly protein. They are comparable to beans in the quality of protein they provide but they are costly calorie-wise. They are very high in fat. Fortunately their fat is unsaturated and does not harm blood vessels.

The nutritive value of nuts and seeds is greatest for children. They are ideal for filling up "bottomless pits." Yes, those peanut butter sandwiches are good for the kids, providing protein, vitamins, minerals, and the calories that a child needs for his growing body.

For adults, however, nuts and seeds must be eaten in moderation. Combining them with vegetables and beans is a good way to include them in your diet. Peanut butter on a thin slice of whole wheat is a perfect pick-me-up. Nuts and seeds provide good, safe fiber. Just remember, they are rich in calories.

There is one nut that is not cholesterol free. The coconut is very high in saturated fat and calories and has been found in experiments to be even more damaging to the arteries than butter and lard. Since coconut oil is widely used in processed foods, it is best to prepare food from scratch as much as possible.

The American Snack

Snacking on the right foods can be a healthy habit. Snacks that are good for you do not have to be tasteless and boring.

Popcorn, for example, is a great fiber source that satisfies the munchies. Air-popped varieties are especially low in calories. Three cups of plain popcorn have only 76 calories.

Vegetable juice is a highly nutritious snack that is low in calories and salt. Low-fat yogurt is a wonderful way to snack and meet your calcium needs.

Have you seen those little mini tuna cans in the supermarket? This great snack is rich in protein, low in calories, and contains omega-3 fish oils that are great for fighting cholesterol.

Bagels have all the goodness of rich pastries without the calories, and they are a good energy source.

Snacking on vegetables, low-fat crackers and cheeses, fruit, and low-sugar, high-fiber cereals are good ways to handle the munchies when they attack.

Peanuts have been a popular snack for Americans since the late 1800s. More than 4 million pounds of them are consumed each day in this country. The best way to eat peanuts and peanut butter is naturally—no salt, no sweeteners.

In fact, studies show that for all the available, most-popular snacks on the market, *unsalted, dry roasted peanuts* are the overall best choice. One ounce of dry roasted, unsalted peanuts contains 160 calories with less than 10 milligrams of sodium, 7 grams of protein, 15 grams of fat, and 5 grams of carbohydrates.

Fruits and Vegetables

Many children grow up with mothers who don't think anything is worth eating unless it's green. How many times a week does a child hear, "Eat your vegetables!"

Unless your child is one of those blessed few who were born loving everything you put before him, then you know what a chore it can be to get a child to eat vegetables and fruit. I know adults who still wait to eat their vegetables after everything else, almost seeming to force them down.

But Mom is right in pushing vegetables and fruits. They are exclusive powerhouses of nutrition and absolutely essential for good health. They fill hungry, young bodies at a much lower cost than Burger City.

Most people like fruits because they are sweet. Because fruits are 80 to 95 percent water, they're refreshing and thirst-quenching—all at a low price calorie-wise and money-wise. What chocolate cream pie can hold its own against a luscious salad of melon, grapes, and other fruits on a hot summer day? Today we can enjoy a variety of fruit all year from our supermarkets.

Fruits contain a low amount of calories in proportion to a large amount of nutrients and vitamins. Fruit, being a great source of fiber, is also a natural laxative. If you eat fruit each day you will never have to worry about constipation.

Fruits are a good summer food. They help replace water lost in the heat and potassium robbed by exercise. Many fruits provide beta-carotene, which is helpful in warding off sun damage to the skin. Exercising in hot weather can cause a person to lose one to two quarts of water per hour.

The more muscle you have, the more water you need. Muscle is 72 percent water. As you become more fit, fresh fruits and water are increasingly beneficial to your health. A banana, orange, and apple each day can give you more than one-half the dietary fiber recommended by the National Cancer Institute.

How Much Is Enough?

How much do we need to eat from the fruit and vegetable categories? Nutritionists say four servings a day. That's not as much as it seems. If you start with juice in the morning, add an orange later on, and end with a potato and salad at supper you have easily met the recommended amount.

Just be sure to eat a fresh source of vitamin C each day. Since vitamin C is easily destroyed in cooking, an uncooked source is best. Some alternatives are one orange or grape-fruit, two tomatoes, two servings of strawberries or melons, and pineapple. Vitamin C is also available in brussels sprouts, cauliflower, and dark-green vegetables like collards, kale, broccoli, turnip greens, asparagus, and squash.

You also need a daily supply of vitamin A. This can be provided through carrots, broccoli, beets, winter squash or pumpkin, and dark-green leafy vegetables like collards, water cress, turnip and mustard greens, yellow corn, tomatoes, cantaloupe, oranges, peaches, and plums. Other vital minerals found in fruits and vegetables are calcium, potassium, and iron.

Fresh fruits and vegetables are best. Frozen should be your next selection. Eat canned only if you have no other choice. Avoid buying those fruits and vegetables packaged in rich, heavy syrups or sauces. If possible, freeze your own fruits and vegetables.

Cut or prepare fresh fruits and vegetables right before serving to prevent nutrient loss. If possible, eat them raw. Cooked vegetables will retain more of their vitamins and minerals if they are microwaved, pressure cooked, or steamed. Boiling in water is the least desirable method of preparation. Crispness should remain in vegetables that are cooked just until tender.

A Pretty Good Deal

If you aren't convinced yet of the importance of fruits and vegetables, maybe the following facts will totally persuade you.

Fiber found in fruits and vegetables has been shown to inhibit the conversion of sugars to fat or triglycerides in the blood. Subjects on a high-sugar diet experienced a 23 percent reduction in triglyceride levels when 18 grams of crude fiber were added to their diets on a daily basis.

Since 1961, studies have shown that pectin, a soluble fiber found in many fruits and a few vegetables, helps lower blood cholesterol. Pectin, the substance that causes jellies and jams to thicken, is most available in apples, grapefruits, grapes, berries, plums, and carrots.

For some reason these high-pectin fruits and vegetables help to decrease the amount of cholesterol the body absorbs from food and increase the amount the body excretes. Heavy doses of fruits and vegetables also reduce the threat of strokes brought on by tiny blood clots in the blood vessels in the brain.

Dark-green and deep-yellow vegetables as well as fruits help protect the body from cancer development. Carotene (vitamin A) helps guard against skin cancer, and cancers of the lung, breast, bladder, and digestive tracts.

Cabbage-type vegetables, like brocolli, cauliflower, cabbage, and turnip greens, actually contain a "cancer-blocking" chemical that protects cells from cancer-causing agents. The risk of cancer in the stomach and large intestine is greatly reduced by including large amounts of these in your diet.

In conclusion, the bulk provided by fruits and vegetables and all fibrous foods will enable you to consume less calories. Eating fruits and vegetables will help to fill you up. They also give you a lot of chewing satisfaction. The water content of these foods also contributes to their filling value. Some studies have indicated that fructose, the number one sugar in fruit, can help suppress the appetite and thereby reduce calorie intake. Sounds like a pretty good deal to me.

11

Supplementing Your Diet

I once read an article by a woman who said she was a professional dieter. Because she knew the calorie count for nearly every food, she considered herself a safe dieter. But during the last six months and the last 25 pounds of her last diet, she suffered with a painful throat infection. "I was living dangerously," she admitted, "because of poor nutrition. I lost weight, but I also lost much of my resistance to infection."

Doctors have found that people recovering from surgery contract infections not because of the surgery but because of poor nutrition. The immune system also does not work right when a person is on an extremely low-calorie diet.

Since statistics show that two out of three people are dieters, you are probably a dieter. Are you endangering your health with a diet that is nutritionally unsound? When you're eating like a horse, you can afford to be more lax in getting all the essential nutrients. If you're a hearty eater, sooner or later enough needed nutrients will be shoveled in with everything else.

But if you are eating like a bird, every morsel counts and becomes critical to your health. When you are down to

1,000 calories or less per day, every bite must be nutritionally sound. Every calorie must carry a nutritional whollop.
You must know if you are giving your body enough
nutrients. That's why you should clear any diet with your
physician before beginning it.

If you are dieting and you smoke or take birth control pills,
your need for balanced nutrition is even greater than that
of other people. The nutrient loss by dieting in combination with these other risks can greatly damage your health.

Female dieters need to be especially careful to include
enough calcium and iron in their diets. Iron deficiency leads
to tiring earlier in the day than is normal, and calcium
deficiency can lead to osteoporosis.

Vital Vitamins

Approximately one-third of the adult American population takes vitamins. The big question is—do they need them?
The answer is, "Yes." If taken wisely, vitamins are very
beneficial, especially to smokers and to the elderly.

Since we are a nation of dieters, many of us do have
minimal vitamin deficiencies. By eating less we supply fewer
nutrients and vitamins to the body. If you consume 2,500
to 3,000 calories of a fairly balanced diet each day, you
probably do not need vitamin supplements.

If you are dieting or consuming less than 2,000 calories
per day, you may be short on some vitamins. Just remember, vitamin supplements alone will not solve your health
problems. Vitamins are just part of a balanced health
program of diet and exercise.

Do you have slow-healing wounds, tiredness, or frequent
illnesses? If your doctor has ruled out any serious health
problems, you may be experiencing vitamin deficiencies. All
pregnant women require vitamin supplements under the
guidance of a physician. Infants and children up to certain
ages require vitamin supplements.

Let's talk about a few of the most vital vitamins.

Vitamin D and Healthy Bones

Vitamin D enhances the body's absorption of calcium and deters osteoporosis. Besides being essential for healthy bones, vitamin D also helps stabilize the nervous system, maintain normal heart function, and normal blood clotting.

If someone cannot be in the sun at least twenty minutes a day, then they should ask their doctor to recommend a dosage and supplement of vitamin D. Eating egg yolks, liver, and tuna will help increase your vitamin D supply.

Until recently vitamin D deficiency and its accompanying rickets was thought to be rare or even eradicated. But in the past few years, the problems have resurfaced, particularly among the elderly. Doctors have difficulty distinguishing osteomalacia (the adult version of rickets) from osteoporosis. Both cause thinning of the bones and can lead to painful deformities.

The best source of vitamin D is still the sun. As we age our bodies manufacture less vitamin D. Older people usually find it harder to digest milk products or may shun them for fear of high cholesterol. Many elderly people are cut off from their best sources of vitamin D—the sun and milk.

The B Vitamins and Stress

For the active person who operates on a tight schedule and deals with daily stress, B vitamin supplements are quite helpful. This family of supplements helps release energy from carbohydrates and fats and helps mobilize protein for the building of new tissue.

You should probably check with your doctor to confirm your need of supplementation and what dosage your body requires. Heavy doses can have side effects as serious as loss of ability to walk.

When prescribed correctly, the B vitamins can be beneficial to health. Vitamin B-6 has been used quite successfully
in treating pinched nerves in the wrist and can help with
other problems of the nervous system. Vitamin B-6 is
thought to be effective in treating pre-menstrual syndrome
(PMS), but the test results are inconclusive.

Riboflavin, a member of the vitamin B complex, can be
found in the following foods: low-fat dairy products, green
leafy vegetables, breads and cereals, organ meats, bananas,
herring, mackerel, crab meat, chicken breast, tuna, and
baked potatoes.

Vitamin C and Old Age

Contrary to what you may have heard, vitamin C will
not prevent or even reduce the number of colds you have,
but it will reduce the severity of them. Vitamin C definitely
helps form collagen and maintain capillaries, bones, and
teeth. This vitamin may be helpful in blocking the formation of cancer-causing nitrosamines. It also helps in the
absorption of iron.

Vitamin C is needed by the enzyme that creates the
connective tissue on which bone-hardening calcium is laid.
Without enough vitamin C, bones cannot make use of
calcium as they should.

A group of British researchers believe that vitamin C can
help slow or even stop bones from becoming weak and
crumbly with age. Their study revealed low levels of
vitamin C in people with hip fractures as compared to those
without fractures—even when hipbone calcium content was
the same.

Severe vitamin C deficiencies are rare. Most Americans get
enough vitamin C without needing supplementation. Mostly
older people who live alone suffer from this deficiency.
Everyone, especially the elderly, needs adequate vitamin C
in their diets for healthy bones.

Be sure to eat foods that are rich in vitamin C daily. These include: citrus fruits, tomatoes, green peppers, strawberries, melons, potatoes, and dark-green vegetables.

Vitamin E and Air Pollution

Vitamin E aids in the formation of red blood cells, muscles, and other tissues, and protects vitamin A and essential fatty acids from oxidation. Vitamin E is known to help the body in the healing process.

Vitamin E may help minimize damage from air pollution and help prevent cancer. Tests done on animals have shown they suffered less lung damage from air pollution when given vitamin E supplements. This vitamin may be especially helpful in minimizing the effects of our diminishing ozone layer—particularly skin cancer.

Because a person rarely experiences a real deficiency of this vitamin, any supplementation should be done with your doctor's knowledge.

Vitamin A and Cancer

Vitamin A is necessary for bone growth and teeth development. It prevents night blindness and helps form and maintain healthy skin, hair, and mucous membranes. Vitamin A may be helpful in the prevention of cancer, but it is not a cure. Studies have shown a lower rate of cancer among those with diets rich in vitamin A.

Beta-carotene, a substance in many fruits and vegetables that the body converts to vitamin A, is thought to be a most promising prospect as an anti-cancer nutrient.

If you take a supplement of this vitamin or any other, do so only with your doctor's advice and consent. Avoid megadoses of any vitamin. You can seriously damage your health by overdosing on certain vitamins.

Iron and Fatigue

Do you have a craving for ice cubes that won't quit? Better check your iron levels. The insatiable desire for ice cubes is called *pagophagia* and is a symptom of iron deficiency. Anemics can chew up as many as ten trays of ice cubes a day. Others constantly chew celery, carrots— anything brittle. Iron deficiency can be cleared up in days, but the damage to teeth from crunching on ice may be permanent.

Iron is a trace mineral that is present in every living cell and helps build strong bodies. We need only a little, but iron is often too low or missing almost entirely in women.

Iron exists in a combined state with protein; its major function is to combine with protein and copper in making hemoglobin, the coloring matter of red blood cells. Hemoglobin transports oxygen in the blood from the lungs to tissues.

Iron builds up blood quality and aids the body in coping with stress and disease. Iron also works with other nutrients to help improve the respiratory system.

In addition to energizing oxygen to the cells, iron carts away oxygen's waste product, carbon dioxide. It supplies power to muscles and helps metabolize glucose. Iron deficiency leaves a person feeling drained.

Iron, because it can be stored in the liver, spleen, bone marrow, and blood, is used over and over again by the body rather than being "used up" like some nutrients. To maintain proper functioning of iron in the body, both calcium and copper are needed in the diet.

Women need more iron during menopause and pregnancy. Increased iron is also needed in case of hemorrhage, rapid growth, or loss of blood. People who exercise need more iron than those who are inactive. The pounding of feet through walking, aerobics, or running can deplete iron.

The most common lack of iron is iron-deficiency anemia, resulting in pale skin, abnormal fatigue, constipation, brittle nails, and difficult breathing. A low iron level leads to early tiring during normal exercise.

Getting the Iron You Need

Cooking in an old-fashioned, cast-iron pan can increase the amount of iron in a food, especially if it is acidic and has a high moisture content. The iron in the cookware actually seeps out into the food during preparation and can be safely used by the body.

One study showed that high-acid, moist foods, such as applesauce and spaghettti sauce, had twenty-six and eight times more iron, respectively, when heated in an iron pan. This gives you 50 percent of the required amounts of iron for one day in the applesauce and 40 percent from the spaghetti sauce.

Take iron supplements only under your doctor's supervision. Excessive, long-term use of iron supplements can cause damage to the liver, spleen, and pancreas and can even kill you.

Rather than relying solely on iron supplements, look to foods that can supply your iron needs: liver and red meats, green leafy vegetables, whole grain cereals and bread, pinto beans, raisins, and broccoli. Iron is found in spinach but is more easily absorbed from other iron-rich vegetables. Eat citrus fruits with iron-rich foods to enhance iron absorption. Eat liver at least once a month.

Copper and Cholesterol

Most Americans do not get enough of this valuable mineral. Sufficient levels of copper can positively influence blood cholesterol, the electric patterns of the heart, and glucose tolerance.

Research over the past ten years has shown that a diet low in copper raises blood cholesterol. When subjects were given the same diet with copper, cholesterol levels dropped. Copper is needed for the efficient functioning of two enzymes that lower cholesterol.

A copper deficiency will also tamper with the heart's electric patterns. Research with mice on high-fat diets in which cardiac damage was detected showed their diets lacked copper. Further research showed that mice with copper-added diets had no heart problems and lived five times longer than those on copper-deleted diets.

Diabetics should be interested to know that low levels of copper in their bodies will hinder glucose tolerance. Copper actually makes insulin work more effectively. Consult your physician before making any self-prescribed changes in your routine or medication.

Copper should come from the foods you eat, not from supplements. Most doctors do not advise the use of copper supplements.

Skim milk enhances the absorption of copper. Good sources of copper include: beef liver, Brazil and cashew nuts, sunflower and pumpkin seeds, oysters, wheat germ, and high-bran cereals.

We need two to three milligrams of copper per day. The biggest dietary enemies of copper are too much zinc, vitamin C, and sugar.

Zinc and Eating Disorders

Zinc can greatly influence the body's ability to grow and resist disease. Research indicates that we become more susceptible to disease as we age because our bodies lose their ability to absorb zinc.

Our bodies need zinc in order to make protein and cells. A zinc deficiency adversely affects the release of stored vitamin A from the liver.

Too little zinc alters the sense of taste and smell. Zinc also seems to influence areas of the brain that control eating and drinking. Animals that were deprived of zinc were also apt to drink alcohol. Without zinc, they actually craved alcohol.

In tests, zinc-deficient animals developed symptoms of anorexia and bulimia. Deprived of zinc, the animals ate less and less. When they did eat, they binged and then threw up their food. Under stress these animals began to eat more than normal. When they received adequate zinc, the animal's eating habits returned to normal.

Studies on bulimic and anorexic women confirmed their zinc deficiencies. How did these women behave? Just as the zinc-deficient animals only with the addition of laxative abuse, induced vomiting, and unnecessary dieting. Zinc also aids the body in determining when it has had enough to eat.

Low zinc will aggravate gum disease brought on by plaque formation. People with gum disease have a zinc deficiency; and research has shown gum disease disappeared when the zinc deficiency was corrected.

Zinc deficiences affect blood sugar. A zinc-dependant enzyme in the liver is located right at the point in glucose metabolism that leads either to energy burning or fat storage. A shortage of zinc causes this enzyme to become inactive, resulting in fat being stored instead of burned. People who say, "Everything I eat turns to fat," should have their zinc level tested.

Oysters, grains, and nuts are rich in zinc. If you take a supplement of zinc, do not exceed 30 milligrams a day without medical supervision.

Potassium and High Blood Pressure

How important is potassium to your body? What does it do for your health? Where do you find it?

High blood pressure is the most important risk factor in the development of a stroke. Sodium is known to adversely affect blood pressure. But do we know how important potassium is in neutralizing the affects of sodium?

Potassium has a protective influence all its own. Hospital studies show that people with a positive potassium-sodium ratio have a reduced likelihood of having high blood pressure. The study found that people are eating roughly about half the potassium they need in their diets.

The best source of potassium (the third most abundant mineral in the body after calcium and phosphorus) is fresh fruit. Cantaloupe, tomatoes, oranges, bananas, and peaches are good sources. Fresh fruit should be eaten with every meal as a protection against stroke.

A low-sodium, high potassium diet will usually help lower blood pressure. So will moderate exercise. Tests show that the best way to tackle high blood pressure is a low-sodium, high-potassium diet coupled with moderate exercise.

If you take diuretics, you may have been told that eating potassium-rich foods will make up for potassium losses. You would have to eat at least four or more potassium-rich bananas each day to make up for the loss of potassium through use of diuretics. Even then, the potassium would be poorly retained by the body and you would be left with the calories. Avoid diuretics if at all possible and drink water instead.

Chromium and Diabetes

Candy, cookies, and all foods high in sugar can lead to a deficiency of the mineral chromium. Chromium is an important nutrient that maintains normal levels of sugars and fats in the blood. A deficiency in this nutrient may lead to diabetes and heart disease.

In a study volunteers drank solutions containing sugar. They measured the levels of insulin, the hormone that helps keep blood sugar on an even keel. They also measured the amount of chromium the volunteers excreted in their urine. They found that sugars cause the body to produce high insulin levels and excrete large amounts of chromium.

Foods high in sugar are usually low in most nutrients, including chromium. Even sugary breakfast cereals are not good. By contrast, fortified, low-sugar breakfast cereals are high in chromium. Chromium can also be found in vegetables, whole grains, and fruits.

Minerals and Your Skin

Minute quantities of trace minerals aid our skin as it works to fight the effects of pollution, emotional stress, and improper skin care. These minerals function by working along with the enzymes in our bodies to create chemical reactions that help to increase the flow of oxygen to the skin, thus encouraging cell turnover.

For example, copper is essential in the formation of skin pigment. Iron produces carbon dioxide and promotes cell renewal. Zinc helps repair skin cells and works to counteract the cellular damaging effects of sunlight. Magnesium helps the skin hold moisture.

When a body is lacking in trace minerals, it shows in the skin through forehead furrows and a dull, lifeless complexion. Trace minerals help the skin renew and repair itself by enabling it to breathe.

Play It Safe

Remember that vitamins and minerals are only part of a balanced diet. Most of your nutrients should come from natural foods that you eat, not from bottles of supplements manufactured by pharmaceutical companies.

Once you begin dieting, you may also be cutting out important nutrients that could endanger your health or lower your resistance to disease. Never try to reduce on a strict diet that requires you to maintain less than a 1,000 calorie per day regimen. If you are on a low-calorie diet, first clear it with your doctor and ask him to recommend a good multi-vitamin.

─── 12 ───

You Can Prevent Osteoporosis

If you are under thirty-five, you may not be too concerned about your calcium intake. But calcium is attracting more and more attention because a growing number of Americans, particularly women, suffer with thinning bones or osteoporosis.

Those most at risk seem to be women over age fifty, slender, fair complexioned, inactive smokers with a family history of the disease. This condition affects one in four women over age sixty.

The loss seems to be greater in women because of female hormones. Menopause causes lower estrogen levels and less calcium to be absorbed from food. When taken with calcium supplements, low doses of the female hormone estrogen seem to slow the process of calcium drain.

The earliest sign of the disease is loss of height. This happens when the weakened bones of the spine become compressed. Later a curving of the spine will become evident. Any minor fall can break a bone. Women often experience no pain until a break occurs.

Most sufferers of osteoporosis have thin back bones that become compressed, causing pain and stooping. Osteoporosis is not so much a disease as a natural decline of the bones due to age. We have our peak bone mass at age thirty-five. If you have a good bone mass at this age, chances are you have good protection against bone deterioration later on.

Osteoporosis is certain when bones have lost 30 to 40 percent of their mineral content. Fractures of the spine, hips, and wrists most commonly occur with osteoporosis. The reason these bones are the first to thin is because they have the greatest amounts of calcium.

A Calcium Crisis?

What's the big deal about calcium? Shouldn't every man, woman, and teenager be getting enough in milk, our all-American drink? Adults often avoid milk because of fat or stomach problems, and teens prefer carbonated beverages. Experts estimate that up to 50 percent of teenage girls, who need extra calcium to support growing bones, get only 600 milligrams a day—about half of the RDA for their age.

Women start losing calcium fairly early in life. To prevent osteoporosis, women need to pack in a reasonable calcium intake after age thirty-five. The RDA is recommending 1,000 milligrams of calcium daily. Right now the average adult woman consumes only 450 to 500 milligrams of calcium per day—just about half of what she needs.

Why is calcium so important to the body? Calcium powers our heartbeat, contracts muscles, and moves fluid in and out of cells. If the body doesn't receive enough calcium from the diet, it extracts calcium from the bones. The body works continually at building bones until age thirty-five when bone loss begins. We must exercise and feed our bones right so we can protect ourselves from having stooped, breakable bones in our old age.

Milk—The Perfect Food?

Milk is as American as apple pie. Naturally loaded with calcium, protein, carbohydrates, and potassium, milk is very often fortified with vitamins A and D as well as iron. No wonder nutritionists sometimes call it nature's perfect food.

Milk is one of our best sources for calcium. Two 8-ounce glasses provide 75 percent of the Recommended Dietary Allowance for an adult. To get the calcium equivalent of one cup of milk, you would have to eat a 10-ounce package of frozen broccoli, two 3.5 ounce servings of salmon, or two 1-ounce servings of canned sardines!

With 8 grams of protein per cup, milk has more protein than a poached egg. One glass also gives you 12 grams of carbohydrates and 370 milligrams of potassium. Fortified milk contains one-third of the RDA for vitamins A and D.

The main sources of calcium for Americans are milk and milk products. For the dieter this comes as bad news. Many dairy products are high in calcium, fat, and cholesterol. Fat may be the single most important reason for the 51 percent drop in popularity of milk over the past two decades. A new, health-conscious public began cutting fat from its diet by discarding whole milk.

Americans are getting a taste for low-fat foods. Many people have found that skim and reduced-fat varieties of milk are excellent alternatives to high-fat whole milk. How much better is skim milk? An 8-ounce glass of skim milk contains only .44 grams of fat and just 86 calories. Skim milk actually contains a little more calcium per serving than whole milk.

What About Lactose Intolerance?

Some people can't drink milk due to a condition called *lactose* intolerance. *Lactase,* the digestive enzyme that breaks down the milk sugar lactose, is missing in their bodies.

All of us are born with lactase in our systems, but approximately 70 percent of us mysteriously lose our lactase supply sometime between the ages of five and twenty. Many of us don't experience symptoms at all. But for some six to ten percent of white Americans and a whopping 70 to 90 percent of blacks, drinking milk may result in stomach pains, gas, and diarrhea.

Lactose-intolerant people don't have to miss out on milk's nutritional value. Some companies now manufacture milk with lactase added. Some lactose-intolerant people can drink milk, but no more than one glass without experiencing problems.

Drinking milk with a meal may also alleviate symptoms for some people. The rate at which lactose enters the system is slowed, which reduces the risk of stomach problems.

Lactose-intolerant people may find it helpful to substitute yogurt for milk or add low-fat cheese to their diets. This way they can obtain adequate calcium without the fat and cholesterol associated with whole milk products.

Calcium is also present in dark green leafy vegetables such as collards, turnip greens, spinach and broccoli, salmon and sardines (eaten with the bones), oysters, and tofu (soybean curd). These sources of calcium are great for people who are lactose intolerant.

Checking Calcium Content

A fairly new test can examine the state of your bones and compare their calcium content to that of an average person of the same age and background. The name of that test is QCT, and it costs between $96 and $142. This simple, fifteen-minute test involves a very slight exposure to radiation.

The test measures the area of bone most sensitive to calcium loss by looking inside the bone. The purpose of the test is to prevent fractures before they occur, which frequently happens when bone loss approaches 40 percent. By age seventy-five, the average person has lost more than 50 percent of their inner bone.

Doctors recommend that a woman entering menopause have this test so that a customized plan to combat and prevent osteoporosis can be designed for her. With the test, the doctor can continue to follow the patient's progress.

The Calcium Connection

Low calcium intake has been linked to high blood pressure and colon cancer. Studies have shown that the greater the consumption of milk products, the less hypertension.

The key is not necessarily how much calcium we consume, but how much we absorb into the blood. Although 99 percent of the calcium is in our bones, it's the remaining 1 percent in the tissue and blood that keeps us alive. This 1 percent is needed for hormones and blood clotting.

Too much or too little calcium can be fatal. That is why our bodies strive so hard to keep the calcium in the blood and tissues at a certain level. If the calcium levels in the blood get too low, the body begins to draw calcium from the intestines, kidneys, and bones. This is the beginning of trouble.

Vitamin D helps the body absorb calcium. Large quantities of protein can lead to loss of calcium through the urine. Most everyone can stand to cut back on their protein intake. For women, 44 grams of protein a day is plenty; for men, 56 grams. One chicken breast has 26 grams of protein; a three-ounce sirloin steak has 20 grams.

Large amounts of phosphorus can also inhibit calcium absorption. But when protein, phosphorus, and calcium are put together in the right quantities, they work like a charm in making the most of the body's calcium. Balance is the key. For example, soft drinks contain phosphorus but no protein or calcium. Large doses of soft drinks can become a real drain on your body's calcium reserves. Magnesium, which is found in fresh green vegetables, helps the body utilize calcium also.

A pint of milk each day will cut the risk of colon cancer. Milk along with fiber, vitamin D, and regular exercise will greatly reduce chances of colon cancer. Studies have shown that men who exercised regularly had 60 percent less colon cancer. Calcium binds with toxic bile acids from the liver, turning them into compounds that can be excreted harmlessly through the colon.

Dancer's Disease

Older, inactive women are not the only victims of osteoporosis. This bone disease can begin as early as twenty years of age in women who don't eat or exercise right. Young dancers who diet excessively have been known to develop osteoporosis.

Those who diet severely enough to affect their menstrual cycles are in danger of developing weak bones for the same reasons women in menopause do. Ballet dancers who don't start menstruating until age 14 or who never get their periods may permanently damage their bones. Exercises that normally strengthen bones apparently aren't enough to offset estrogen loss. What is so heartbreaking for these young dancers is that the damage seems to be permanent.

Eat Your Way to Strong Bones

New calcium-enriched foods on the market and more knowledge about bone disease makes it possible for you to eat your way to stronger bones.

Such calcium-rich foods as broccoli, low-fat cheese, collards, milk, raw oysters, tofu, and yogurt are quite helpful. One cup of broccoli, collards, mustard or turnip greens, or kale (cooked) provide at least 100 milligrams of calcium at less than 50 calories. Also low in calories are mozzarella or provolone cheeses—an ounce contains more than 100 milligrams of calcium at about 100 calories. Canned sardines (with the bones) have an excellent supply of calcium with few calories.

Skim milk is so much better for adults than whole milk. Recent research has shown that drinking two glasses of skim milk each day can actually prolong your life. This often-shunned drink can actually reduce the body's serum cholesterol levels.

The secret seems to lie in the tendency of skim milk to increase the amount of high-density lipoproteins (HDL) in the body. HDL protects against heart disease by preventing fat build-up in the arteries. HDL may be nature's perfect way to wash and scrub clogged or potentially clogged arteries.

Skim milk is best; 1 percent is better; 2 percent is okay. But, remember that 1 and 2 percent mean that 1 or 2 percent of the total weight of that container of milk is fat. If you're interested in losing weight, you will want to know that 36 percent of the calories in a container of 2 percent milk will come from that 2 percent of fat. Many doctors recommend 2 percent for children over the age of two. But for adults, skim is best.

What About Calcium Supplements?

The average woman would have to drink too much milk each day in order to get enough calcium. That's why supplements make sense. Studies have shown that taking a calcium supplement of 1,000 milligrams a day can slow the calcium depletion, but will not prevent it. Before age thirty-five, supplements can assist in the formation of strong, dense bones.

My doctor advised me to take my calcium supplement at bedtime because calcium is stored during the day and lost at night when it leaves the bones in order to maintain that all-important blood level. At night when no food is being taken in, the bones are the body's only source of calcium. Calcium at night will help the blood levels stay normal and eliminate the drain on the bones.

Don't take calcium supplements on an empty stomach. Take it with milk or yogurt. These products will help you get the maximum benefit from your supplement. My doctor also advised me to take the calcium supplements that are labeled "calcium carbonate" because they are much easier to digest.

No More Brittle Bones

Regular exercise is an important part of preventing and treating osteoporosis. Exercises that place moderate stress on the spine and the long bones of the body, such as walking, jogging, dancing, and bicycle riding are good.

Since bone is a living tissue, activity helps bone tissue hang on to its calcium. When the body is inactive, the bones are more easily depleted of calcium. Without exercise the astronauts lost 5 percent of their bone mass each day.

Some reports indicate that walking improves bone condition just as well as calcium supplements or estrogen. Other studies have revealed that women who exercise regularly have no bone loss while those who are inactive regularly lose bone.

I came across a study done on people suffering from osteoporosis. It showed that they benefitted from a floor exercise called the "mad cat." The "mad cat" exercise involves getting on your hands and knees and humping your back up as high as you can and then swaying your back as you lower your tummy toward the floor.

This exercise actually strengthens the muscles that attach to the vertebrae and slows the loss of bone mineral mass from the bones. Osteoporosis sufferers who did this back-strengthening exercise had one-third the spinal fractures of sufferers who did not do the exercise. Muscles that pull directly on the bones can strengthen the bones.

If your doctor says you have osteoporosis, then estrogen, calcium supplements, and exercise will benefit you.

A dosage of 1,000 milligrams per day and an exercise program of walking, jogging, or climbing stairs (any exercise that stresses the bones of the pelvis and spine) for 55 minutes, three times per week has been shown to actively increase bone mass by an average of 4 percent. Osteoporosis is a treatable and preventable disease.

13
Drink To Your Health

Our bodies can go for weeks without food but only a couple of days without water. That's because we are two-thirds water, and water is used in all body functions. Water is the most important and probably the most neglected nutrient of all. We often pay more attention to our vitamin and mineral needs than we do our water needs.

Without water, life would be impossible. Water is a solvent for most other nutrients; a waterway from one part of the body to another for nutrients and metabolic waste products; a necessary digestive aid; and a very important factor in the energy and heat balance of our bodies.

Water cleanses the body of toxins and allows the liver and kidneys to perform more efficiently. Water flushes out excess salt, improves muscle tone, and gives skin a more youthful firmness.

How Much Water Do You Need?

We obtain water from three sources. The first is the fluid we drink. The second source is the food we eat. Virtually all foods contain some water—even meats contain water.

The third source is the water formed in our bodies. This comes from the metabolism of protein, fat, and carbohydrates. One hundred calories of carbohydrate provides 15 grams (about one tablespoon) of water. One hundred calories of fat provides 12 grams of water, and 100 calories of protein provides 10 grams of water.

The average person needs two to three quarts of water each day. Since 40 percent comes from food and metabolism, the amount you have to drink is roughly six, 8-ounce glasses. In a hot environment your body will need even more.

Unfortunately, we drink liquids that actually draw water from the cells. For example, too much alcohol, caffeine, fat, sugar, or salt can lead to dehydrated cells that do not function well. The heart works harder and the body becomes stressed. Too much sodium in your diet causes your body to dilute it by drawing water from the cells. Dehydrated cells don't function correctly.

Excess fluid in the brain cells causes depression and anxiety. But adequate water each day can alleviate these problems and many times totally correct them.

Flooding Out Fat

Did you know that water is the least expensive, least harmful, and most effective appetite suppressant available? An increase in water intake can actually reduce fat deposits while a decrease in water consumption will result in an increase in fat deposits. How does this happen?

First, the kidneys cannot function properly without adequate water. If they aren't able to do their job, they dump some of their load onto the liver. Since one of the major jobs of the liver is to metabolize fat into usable energy, it cannot metabolize as much fat if it must do some of the kidneys' work. Since more fat remains in storage, weight loss comes to a standstill.

Too often we reach for food when we actually are hungry for water. If you can establish a habit of drinking water throughout the day, your body will start calling for water regularly and you will find yourself eating less.

But Won't I Retain Fluid?

Many dieters have the mistaken notion that drinking lots of water will only make them more bloated and puffy. Actually just the opposite is true. An inadequate supply of water triggers survival mechanisms that cause the body to hoard every drop of available water in extracellular spaces—creating swollen feet, legs, and hands. The more water you drink, the less fluid your body retains.

Diuretics in no way address the real problem of fluid retention, which is an inadequate water supply. Water pills that guarantee weight loss force out stored water along with all the nutrients this water comes in contact with.

But nothing has changed as far as the brain and body are concerned. Survival is still threatened, and the body still works furiously to store water. Usually the lost water is quickly replaced. Only when you consume plenty of water will your body release its stored water.

If excess salt is to blame for your fluid retention problems, drinking plenty of water and cutting back on salt will help. Water washes away salt.

Once your body becomes accustomed to proper intake of water, you will notice your machine is running more smoothly; your fat is being metabolized instead of stored (you aren't gaining weight); you actually begin to thirst for water; and your hunger decreases.

Dangers of Dehydration

Did you know your body is losing water every minute of the day and night? When you breathe, expired air is always saturated with water vapor. You may lose half a quart of water per day this way, even when you don't exercise or work strenuously. That same amount normally evaporates through your skin on a daily basis. This is called *insensible perspiration,* which is part of your body's mechanism to maintain and control a constant body temperature.

A person cannot skip drinking water one day and then compensate for it the next day by drinking twice as much. Your intake of water should be kept on an even, daily basis. To maintain a correct fluid balance, you should drink water throughout the day, everyday.

Symptoms of dehydration include feeling weak, light-headed, flushed, intolerant of heat, irritable, or confused. Athletes will notice their performance lagging or their muscles cramping as they approach dehydration.

Most of the time when we approach dehydration, our bodies respond. Brain cells sense a drop in blood volume and an increase in the salt levels of the blood. The brain excretes a biochemical that makes us thirsty. At the same time the kidneys conserve water, and we urinate a darker, more concentrated fluid.

In healthy young people, this system works great in keeping the right amount of water in our bodies. We drink what we need and if we overdrink, the kidneys dump the excess.

But some people must drink more than what their thirst calls for. People who are prone to kidney stones are advised to drink more water. This reduces the formation of stones, and water dilutes the minerals that crystalize in the kidneys to form stones.

What Causes Dehydration?

Three conditions that can bring on dehydration are common medications, normal aging, and summer heat.

If the label on a medication says to drink plenty of fluids, make sure you do. Drinking plenty of water with a medicine allows your body to absorb more of it.

Some doctors prescribe diuretics for edema, but once the swelling goes down patients often continue taking their medication. This is dangerous and can result in dehydration. Once the edema is gone, the dosage should be decreased by your doctor.

Research has shown that our thirst mechanisms slow with age. Healthy older people whose bodies need water are not likely to feel thirsty the way young people do. As we grow older our bodies will not automatically call for water. We have to train ourselves to drink water.

As we age, we begin to lose water from our cells just as we lose muscle. Just as exercise compensates for muscle loss, water prevents fluid retention and loss of water from the cells.

Diabetes can cause dehydration in older people. The kidneys use up lots of water to filter sugar out of the blood. The younger diabetic will experience great thirst, but the older diabetic may not. The body overheats when it lacks water, causing the blood volume to drop. A person can dry up and die as the body draws water out of the cells to restore the blood volume and cool itself.

If you live in or visit a hot, dry climate, your water needs will be greater than those living in a moist, cooler climate.

Water and Exercise

Replacing the water you lose during exercise will keep the body's cooling system functioning. Hot weather can unexpectedly cause dehydration. During exercise you cannot count on your thirst mechanism to tell you when you need water.

You should drink before, during, and after workouts to be sure you're getting enough. Drink up to 20 ounces an hour or two before exercising. Cold water will be absorbed more quickly by the body. What about Gatorade? Those drinks advertised by athletes are all right, but in no way do they measures up to what water can do for you.

Be aware of your body as you exercise. If exhaustion or weakness begins, avoid dehydration by drinking regularly. The amount you drink depends on the intensity of your exercise, the temperature, and the humidity. If you are overweight, you need more water than a thin person. The more you exercise, the more water you need.

If you are tired and listless after your regular exercise routine, your water intake could be inadequate. The first forty-five minutes after any workout are critical for water replacement. After two hours, it may be too late to avoid the muscle soreness, fatigue, and listlessness that comes from loss of body fluids.

Body fluids are lost through sweating and through exhalation. On a hot day, you can lose from 2 to 4 percent of your body weight through intense exercise. This translates into one to two and one-half quarts of fluid for a 120-pound woman.

Water helps maintain proper muscle tone. Drinking sufficiently gives the muscles their natural ability to contract and prevents dehydration. Water also helps prevent sagging skin that follows weight loss. People who lose weight just hate the sagging skin that often follows, so their best means of prevention is to drink plenty of water as they diet and exercise back to health.

Increasing Your Water Intake

Some people tell me they don't like the taste of water, so they just don't drink it. As far as your health and your body are concerned, there can be no substitute for water.

If you don't like water, begin by drinking three or four glasses a day and work up gradually to eight or ten. Once you reach eight or ten glasses a day, stick with it.

Never count coffee, tea, or colas as water equivalents. You will find that you drink less of these other liquids anyway as you become "addicted" to water. You will also become addicted to the regularity in bowel movements and to the sense of well-being that an adequate water supply can give you.

If we could just "tank up" on water we would enjoy better health. Because we cannot store water in our bodies, inadequate intake affects us very rapidly. Even though we can live without food for several days, we could only survive for two days in a hot climate without water.

If you can't stand the taste, try your water with a twist of orange juice or lemon juice. Keep water in the refrigerator since cold water is tastier and more readily absorbed by the body. Drinking from a container in the refrigerator will also help you keep track of your water consumption.

Water is the perfect diet drink. No calories—not even one. Never think that tea, coffee, and juice are substitutes for water. They do not count. When it comes to meeting the body's needs, nothing can beat water.

The Caffeine Buzz

Have you ever tried to get started in the morning without a cup of coffee? If you are like 80 percent of the American public, you get out of bed and head straight for your coffee pot. If an alien from another planet visited earth, he might wonder if caffeine is as essential to life as air and water. Those of us who find it hard to get started without our morning caffeine buzz might also wonder.

Caffeine is a drug found in more than sixty species of plants, including coffee, tea, cocoa, and kola nuts. After being extracted from these sources and powdered, caffeine is added to many popular beverages. Caffeine also doubles as a flavoring agent in baked goods, desserts, and puddings. Children, because of their smaller size, can consume the equivalent of an adult's two to three cups of coffee a day in their caffeinated soft drinks alone.

Caffeine increases alertness and motor performance, decreases fatigue, suppresses appetite, and keeps us awake during situations when we can't afford to fall asleep. Because caffeine is a stimulant, it is added to more than 1,000 nonprescription drugs including diet pills, various stay-awake pills, cold tablets, allergy medicine, and some aspirin products.

Coffee stimulates the central nervous system and acts directly on certain neurotransmitters. Caffeine can increase your heart rate and your basal metabolism, cause secretion of stomach acid, increase urine production, dilate some blood vessels and constrict others. Our bodies quickly absorb and rapidly distribute caffeine throughout the body. However, the less food in your stomach, the faster caffeine will be absorbed.

How Much Is Safe?

For years the U.S. Food and Drug Administration has considered caffeine to be "generally recognized as safe," but that official rating was changed in 1980. Recent research associates caffeine-containing beverages with heart disease, pancreatic cancer, and fibrocystic breast disease. Is the "perk" worth it or are we setting ourselves up for serious health problems?

Unfortunately, we just don't know for sure because reports and studies do not always agree. Some researchers use real daily coffee drinkers while other studies employ volunteers who occasionally drink a large dose. Other variables like tobacco or alcohol intake were not always well controlled and may distort the results.

How much caffeine can you consume in one day without inviting problems? Experiencing harmful side effects depends on your weight, sex, age, fitness level, and metabolic or medical problems. How and when you consume your coffee also makes a difference. Drinking black coffee on an empty stomach at breakfast will give you higher blood levels of caffeine faster than an after-dinner coffee with cream. The experts recommend you limit coffee to not over two to three cups a day.

Remember that caffeine is a drug and any drug taken in excess can be dangerous. The lethal dose of caffeine in humans is five to ten grams or seventy-five cups of coffee consumed in one sitting. An overdose of that amount will result in death from convulsive heartbeats. Anyone with a history of irregular heartbeats should consider avoiding caffeine entirely.

Studies claim that drinking eight to ten cups a day (or for some two to three) is a strong sign of "caffeinism," a condition in which the body requires caffeine to continue normal functioning. How can you test for this caffeine addiction? Chronic users of caffeine typically develop a headache sixteen hours after the last dose, which is alleviated by drinking more caffeine. If you can drink coffee all day and into the night and still fall asleep, you have the habit.

Helpful or Harmful?

While caffeine can relieve headaches by acting as a vasodilator to open blood vessels of the brain, it also can constrict blood vessels to the heart and raise blood pressure. Drinking coffee in the morning to prevent dizziness and fainting may be beneficial to those with low blood pressure. That same advice, however, can be harmful to the high blood pressure sufferer.

Does coffee give you ulcers? Coffee increases the flow of stomach acid, thus irritating an already existing ulcer or inflamed stomach lining. Research does not prove that coffee leads to ulcers, although people with ulcers will probably experience discomfort by drinking black coffee, which is very acidic on an empty stomach.

In experiments with laboratory animals, large doses of caffeine produced birth defects like missing fingers and toes. Since no human studies have been done, the extent of damage to human babies by caffeine is undetermined. Since caffeine is a drug that affects the nervous system, it should be eliminated if you are pregnant or breast-feeding.

A recent study showed that freshly-brewed coffee can reduce blood flow to the brain by 25 percent. There is a link between blood flow to the brain and brain functions such as memory, ability to concentrate, and motor skills. How therefore can coffee make anyone think better and achieve more?

Drawbacks to Caffeine

An athlete can use a caffeinated drink before workouts to maximize the release of fat into the bloodstream for more energy. But that same caffeine can deposit fatty acids in the heart and arteries of the inactive person.

Caffeine is much like an amphetamine and causes a hyper feeling that makes relaxing difficult. Withdrawal from caffeine causes irritability and fatigue. If you drink six or more cups a day and experience withdrawal symptoms when deprived of your usual amount, you probably are abusing coffee and need to cut back.

While coffee and tea can speed up your metabolism and increase the burning of calories, they can also lower blood sugar and increase the return of hunger sensations. I suggest no more than two cups of caffeinated drinks per day.

I have found the decaffeinated coffees and teas to be just as tasty as the caffeinated. Some decaffeinated coffees contain methylene chloride, a suspected carcinogen. Read the label carefully before you buy decaffeinated coffee. Drink those whose labels show an absence of this substance.

As for herb teas, I suggest moderation and variety. Since herbal teas can also contain some dangerous chemicals, it is best to limit your consumption of them and make sure you drink only freshly brewed teas.

Guess What You're Losing

Recent studies indicate that coffee and tea consumption reduces the absorption of iron by the body. The *American Journal of Clinical Nutrition* reported that a normally-brewed cup of coffee reduces the iron absorption from a hamburger by 39 percent. A cup of tea decreases the iron absorption by 64 percent. This effect occurs up to one hour after a meal.

Did you know that coffee can sap calcium from your body? One study measured calcium loss by the amount of calcium excreted in the urine of 135 people after they drank regular coffee. For every 300 milligrams of caffeine (two to three cups of coffee), approximately 30 milligrams of calcium were lost. This was twice the amount lost after drinking decaffeinated coffee.

People who consume a lot of caffeine are probably not getting enough calcium. The more caffeine consumed, the more calcium lost. If you rarely eat dairy products, you can deplete your calcium supply with just one cup of regular coffee a day. Older people, in particular, should be careful.

If you cannot give up coffee, then by all means add milk to it. Three tablespoons of milk contain 54 milligrams of calcium, which will more than offset the losses triggered by caffeine.

By the way, how do you like your coffee? If you use a powdered coffee creamer because you think it's less fattening, you'd better check the label. Coffee creamers commonly use coconut oil, which has more saturated fat than pure cream. Each teaspoon of powdered coffee creamer made from coconut oil contains almost two grams of saturated fat. Skim milk is a far better way to lighten your coffee.

Sodas Are No Substitute

When given the choice of milk, coffee, tea, alcoholic beverage, fruit juice, or soft drink, one out of eleven consumers chose a soft drink in 1950. That figure is now three out of eleven. In 1984, soft drinks replaced water as the most-consumed drink in America for the first time. Now Americans average nearly 140 gallons of soft drinks per person per year.

Why such an increase? People don't drink as much milk and coffee due to health reasons. We've been bombarded by advertising that associates carbonated beverages with happiness and youth. Soft drinks are also promoted at fast food restaurants.

Diet sodas have become extremely popular in our weight-conscience society. Market researchers predict that diet sodas will constitute 30 to 40 percent of soda sales by 1990.

Since people insist on drinking carbonated beverages, let's see what they're doing to their bodies. Both diet and regular sodas contain sodium, which aggravates fluid retention and bloating. Both enhance the body's craving for sweets.

Diet sodas contain phosphates, which interfere with the body's ability to absorb calcium. I have received letters from registered nurses and others telling me that they drank so many sodas—mostly diet sodas—that they eventually developed depression, headaches, and nervous problems. After dropping sodas from their diets the problems disappeared. Sodas and diet sodas contain potentially dangerous chemicals and little nutritive value.

As for alcoholic beverages, I see little benefit in drinking them either. A person who has a difficulty controlling his appetite usually loses his grip more easily when consuming alcohol with a meal. Alcoholic beverages are also high in calories.

When You're Thirsty

Juices are good, and fresh is always best. If you can't drink juice as is, mix it half and half with club soda. Juices are always preferable to carbonated beverages that may contain only a small percentage of real fruit juice.

The next time you're thirsty, think it over. Coffee, tea, sodas, and alcohol do little to benefit your body. Reach for a cold, clear glass of water or a nutritious juice drink. You'll be glad you did.

14

Kids and Food

American children who are overweight have increased more than 50 percent over two decades, and our nation is facing an "epidemic of childhood obesity" according to a recent survey. One study found that from 1963 to 1980 there was a 54 percent increase in the prevalence of obesity among children ages six to eleven and a 39 percent rise among adolescents ages twelve to seventeen.

When our children and teens are overweight, we can expect an inevitable rise in adult obesity. A child who enters adolescence obese has one to four odds against ever enjoying normal body weight. If that same child is still obese at the end of his teen years, the chances are one to twenty-eight against him ever reversing his weight problem.

Those who were slender during childhood can more easily lose weight than those who have had a lifelong battle with obesity. Achieving normal body weight and keeping it *is* possible for the overweight child, but it requires effort.

Helping The Overweight Child

Parents must help children learn to control their weight because the fat cells they gain during childhood and adolescence will be with them forever. The overweight child or adolescent will always be battling the bulge because his abundance of fat cells will always make gaining weight easy.

Young children learn habits that set the pattern for their adult behavior. If we foster healthy attitudes and habits in our children, they will more likely maintain those habits in adulthood. The Scriptures admonish parents to "train a child in the way he should go, and when he is old he will not turn from it" (Proverbs 22:6, NIV).

Children unconsciously pattern their lifestyles after their parents. When both mother and father are overweight, a child has an 80 percent chance of also becoming obese. With one overweight parent the risk drops to 40 percent. But this pre-programming, whether genetic, environmental, or a combination of the two, *can* be overcome.

Medical researchers believe our preference for certain foods is largely a matter of habit. Adults who crave fatty foods were probably raised on high-fat diets. Adults who reach for a piece of fruit rather than a candy bar probably grew up without sugary snacks.

Good eating habits are as easy to establish with your children as bad ones. By conditioning your children to prefer a healthful diet, you are helping them establish lifelong patterns that can decrease their risk of heart disease, stroke, and other obesity-related illnesses.

The American Heart Association recommends a doctor-supervised, low-fat, low-cholesterol diet for all children over age two because of ample proof that such a diet leads to better health. Researchers believe the incidence of heart disease has dropped in the past thirty years because of the increase in aerobic exercise and a decrease in fat and cholesterol intake.

Clean Your Plate?

Parents need to watch their own behavior and eating habits. If you eat a balanced, sensible diet coupled with regular exercise that you enjoy, your child will follow your example. Use good, common sense in all you do. Remember, you can get fat on a proper diet as well as on junk or fat foods. Moderation is the key to successful weight control.

The apostle Paul exhorts Christians to "Let your moderation be known unto all men. The Lord is at hand" (Philippians 4:5, KJV). Webster defines moderation as "bringing within bounds. . . avoidance of excess and extremes."

One way to help your child practice moderation in eating is to give him plenty of water between meals. This natural appetite suppressant should cut down on in-between-meal snacking and provide your child with innumerable health benefits.

Parents should also insist that children use utensils, eat slowly, and don't cram food into their mouths. Eating slowly gives the brain time to let the rest of the body know when it has been satisfied. Eating meals at the table instead of in front of the TV will also prevent overindulging.

Some mothers may not agree, but I *never* believe in making a child clean his plate. Your insistence only encourages him to overeat. How can you really know how much he needs at a given time? His body is perfectly capable of telling him when he is full.

If you are having your child regularly checked by a doctor and if his blood, height, and weight are normal, then put reasonable portions of good food before him and let him judge when he is full. Unless he is filling up on sweet, in-between-meal snacks, he will eat enough food each meal.

If Your Child is Overweight

If your child is battling a weight problem, help him look his best. Giving him good hairstyles and nice, attractive clothes within your budget will help maintain his very fragile self-esteem in the face of his weight problem. In fact, a lack of self-esteem could be one reason he overeats. Help him feel good about himself by complimenting his appearance. A child needs to know he is loved no matter what, so remember to remind him how very special he is to you.

Avoid discussing your child's weight with other people in front of him. *Never* tell a child he is getting fat. Such statements only serve to trigger eating disorders. Children can become so fat conscious that they develop what is called "fear-of-fatness-syndrome." Such a child may end up eating a diet so low in fat that his health and normal physical and mental development is jeopardized.

Once a woman mentioned to my daughter that she was gaining weight. She did not even mean to imply that Leah was fat, but to a child such comments can be traumatic. Leah was devastated. She went home and cried. Ignorance and insensitivity can shatter a child's fragile self-esteem.

Children under pressure about weight will often develop bulimia, which is defined as a "continuous, abnormal hunger." They might begin eating binges followed by starvation, which causes serious health and developmental problems. Don't allow your child to get caught up in a preoccupation with thinness.

Children and Diets

Unless excessively overweight, your child doesn't even need to be on a diet. Children and teenagers should diet only under the close supervision of their doctor.

If your physician recommends a diet for your child, let him help plan meals and shop for food. You can make his nutritional regimen more bearable and even fun.

Forget fad diets and spas for an overweight child. They are totally wrong for children. A radical diet can interfere with normal growth and development. If your child is just plump, leave him alone unless his doctor recommends weight loss.

Don't use food as a reward either. If your child has a good

report card, reward him with praise, encouragement, and perhaps a gift of money—but not food.

Do not push your child into an exercise "program" of any kind other than that provided by your school. Aerobics and weightlifting, for example, can even be harmful when performed at too early an age.

You can help your child stay fit by preparing him a balanced diet and seeing that he has plenty of fun, physical activity. If you provide this, as he grows up, your child's weight will adjust and the "baby fat" will disappear.

Why Children Overeat

Why do children overeat? One of the main contributing factors to overeating in children is television. Too many children are having to meet their needs for love, comfort, and companionship from the TV set. When a child's emotional needs are not being met by their parents, the TV and food become surrogate parents.

Even good parents can fall into the habit of substituting the TV and food for their time and attention. If your child is bored, *you* do something with him—don't hand him a bag of chips and turn on the TV. He'd much rather take a walk with you than have all the candy and TV in the world.

Research has shown that children ages six to eleven watch an average of twenty-four hours of TV per week. The more time spent in front of the TV during these years, the more likely a child will become an overweight teen and adult.

TV and snacks go together. When your child is eating and watching TV, absolutely nothing physical is going on except the manufacturing of new fat cells.

Children who watch a lot of TV also tend to have poor grades in school. Why not limit television time and reward children for staying within the boundaries?

Similar research has shown that only 10 percent of teens who watch one hour of TV per day are obese while

20 percent of those who watch five hours or more per day are obese. Studies show that three-fourths of all obese teens become obese adults.

Children and teens, like adults, need physical activity for their mental and physical well-being. Exercise with your child. Play with him. You will be surprised at how his interest in food and TV will instantly wane if he has you and your attention.

Teens and Food

With teens it is important not to let them develop the attitude that food is bad. Teenagers should be able to regard food as a friend. A reluctance to eat or a fear of food can lead to several food disorders and health problems.

To help your family see food as a friend, provide them with balanced low-fat diets. Make mealtime relaxing and enjoyable— not rushed and stressful. Never take care of discipline problems during meals. Studies show people eat more and faster when under stress.

To avoid having a teen who is preoccupied with his weight, say as little as possible about his actual size. A parent's job is to provide the proper encouragement to exercise and eat healthy, balanced meals. If you eat and exercise right, he will almost unconsciously follow your example. Studies have shown that if a parent becomes too involved in trying to make a child lose weight, the child or teen will only eat more.

Every member of your family will benefit if you discourage eating after the evening meal. Heavy bedtime snacks can really pile on the pounds.

Kids can learn to love foods that are good for them and even come to prefer them over their former sweet and fat diets. If it's all they are served, children can acquire a taste for water, salads, vegetables, and fruits. Your kids can even learn to dislike sweets.

Since childhood obesity is directly linked to high blood cholesterol and heart disease, why not give your child the gift of life and help him eat and exercise right? He can't do it without you.

What Does a Growing Child Need?

Let's look at the other side of food-related problems. Why would a twelve-year-old girl be no taller or heavier than she was last year, and medical tests don't show any hormonal or physical problem? When her parents are questioned about the child's diet, they respond, "What? She has a perfect diet. She eats what we eat—a diet low in fat, sugar, and cholesterol with lots of complex carbohydrates."

Young people from such diet-conscious families seem to feel fat is unattractive. Fearful of becoming overweight, these kids don't eat or grow properly.

On the average, children grow two inches per year. If a child is showing little or no growth, then a diet problem may exist. A child who is excessively concerned with how much she weighs or who is always counting calories could be headed for trouble.

We are not talking about adolescent rebellion. No, these children are eating exactly what they have been told to eat. They are good students and high achievers. They are so pitifully attuned to what is "in" that they are bridling the most important part of their formative years—their own growth.

The perfect diet for an adult can be the worst possible diet for a growing child. A pattern of voluntary food restriction in children, if unchecked, can turn into a full-blown eating disorder. The years of critical growth are ages ten to fourteen for boys and eleven to fifteen for girls.

In order to grow properly, a child must eat properly. In studies where children did not receive enough calories in their diets, their growth slowed. Today many doctors are having to teach kids and their parents that eating enough calories in order to grow properly will not make a child fat.

What is the proper diet for a growing boy or girl? In general, adolescents should eat 2,500 to 3,000 calories daily. If a youngster participates in several sports or is extremely active, he may require as many as 3,500 to 4,000 calories per day.

Are You Starving Your Child?

Although a low-fat, high-complex carbohydrate diet is great for reducing the risks of heart disease and other serious ailments in adults, it can do serious harm to a youngster.

Today many affluent, health-conscious parents are actually doing their children more harm than good by insisting they follow a rigid low-fat diet. Some children have been known to develop "failure-to-thrive syndrome" as a result of poor nutrition.

Children who have been on a low-fat diet since infancy become dangerously thin and malnourished. Once these children are fed a normal diet with no restrictions regarding calories, they begin growing and putting on weight.

How could this happen in such a well-fed, health-conscious society and among the well-to-do? Motivated by good intentions, parents unknowingly put their children on diets that are designed strictly for adults. They eliminate sugar, cut back on fat intake, push fruits and vegetables, and give them skim milk to drink. But these good intentions can starve a young child to death.

Growing youngsters need more calories than adults, and they need a certain amount of fat in their diet. Children, for example, should drink whole milk, especially infants and toddlers. For children under two years of age, a low-fat diet is dangerous. Unless carefully regulated by a physician, a restricted diet can be harmful to any growing child.

Before one year of age, nearly all the fatty acids essential to normal body growth and maintenance come from milk.

Breast milk, nature's baby food, is high in fat. Feeding a baby skim milk is unnatural and will cause serious health and growth problems. If you feel your child is overweight, check with your doctor before making any dietary changes or cut-backs in fat. Just to be safe, let your doctor decide what is best for your child.

Encouraging Exercise

Children will by nature get enough exercise if you encourage them and provide the right setting. A gym set in the yard with climbing bars and swings will provide hours of fun and body-building exercise. Family ball games, school sports, and swimming are also good. Keep activity-inducing toys like jump ropes and soccer balls handy.

Take walks with your children as often as possible. They will absolutely love your attention, and both of you will benefit from the exercise. Perhaps the whole family could walk together two or three evenings a week.

Children need a lot of variety in exercise. Their attention spans are short, and they do best at their own pace, going from one activity to another. Youngsters are turned off by activities that take up too much time or are too repetitive.

Parents should reward children for any regular physical activity that will help them stay fit. For example, if your child rides his bike regularly, a new bike horn or mirror would encourage him in that activity.

Dumb Jocks or High Achievers?

Remember hearing the term, "dumb jocks"? Well that is a myth. Evidence shows that students who participate in athletics actually perform better in school. One study of university students revealed that the grade point average of students involved in athletics is generally higher than those who don't participate. While more research is needed in this area, it is obvious that fitness helps students and adults maximize their mental capabilities.

Other studies have revealed that those who become fit are more self-sufficient and stable. As self-esteem improves, so does performance in school or on the job. Even in young children the stimulus of exercise brings on rapid growth and mental advancement ahead of those who do not exercise.

Teachers will tell you that when children return from an exercise class, they are in a better frame of mind to learn. Physical activity does not make children more intelligent, it just makes them more receptive to what is being taught.

Exercise teaches self-discipline that can be applied to all areas of life. Problems arise only when more attention is given to exercise than to learning, and the "dumb jock" routine begins. Exercise must be done in moderation.

Coping With Childhood Stress

Stress is routine for most adults. In fact, it is so routine that sometimes we forget that our children are experiencing stress as well. If we do realize they're under pressure, too often we try to shield them from it.

"Is that so bad?" you might ask. Sometimes it is. Moderate stress is actually healthy and can even add spice and challenge to life. Besides, how will your child learn how to deal with stress unless he learns it from you?

Discourage your child from turning to food to cope with stress. You may have unwittingly fostered this behavior in your child. When was the last time you treated your son or daughter to a milkshake for being good at the doctor's office? Do you resort to food for comforting their bumps, bruises, and skinned knees? Instead, substitute non-food rewards by giving them plenty of your time, love, comfort, and affection.

Here are some more suggestions on how to help your child cope with stress.

1. Discover the areas of stress in your child's life and determine if any of them should be avoided. For example, if too many activities at school prevent him from keeping up with his homework, then determine which activities should be dropped.

2. If grades and schoolwork are stressful, help you child develop good study habits. Provide him with a special, quiet, well-lighted place to study. Help him organize his work and learn to make notes of projects and due dates. Offer rewards for jobs well-done and for effort put forth.

Notice I didn't say reward your child for making A's. An average grade might be just as good for one child as an "A" would be for another. You have to know your child's capabilities and work within that framework, or you will only increase his stress. By helping him promptly complete assignments, you will encourage him to deal with stress through organization and strategy. He will soon develop a sense of accomplishment and mastery over stressful situations.

3. Don't expect your child to be an adult. He is, after all, a child. Take time to view life from the perspective of a toddler who must be juggled between sitters while mom works, the new kid in school who just moved from another state, or an impressionable teen who is being pressured by her peers. Understanding, not anger, will help your child cope with the stresses of growing up.

There are three types of stress: unavoidable, avoidable and necessary. *Unavoidable stress,* like a death in the family or serious illness, can be dealt with by encouraging the child to talk about his feelings and by pointing him to the help that is available through prayer and God's Word.

Avoidable stress can come from adults or other children. Sometimes teachers can unintentionally hurt a child. If your child is overweight, teasing from other children can be stressful and should not be allowed to continue. In these cases, get to the bottom of the matter and try to see that it never occurs again.

Necessary stress helps build character and confidence. If you've laid down the law that no one goes outside to play if bedrooms are not in order, your kids need to know you mean business. Teaching your child to effectively handle his homework and chores at home is sometimes stressful, but the rewards are worth the trouble.

The last thing you want is for your child to see food as a stress reliever. Teach him or her how to go to the Lord when they are facing problems or pressure situations.

15

Beverly's Low-Fat Diet

People often ask me, "Beverly, what do *you* eat?" In this chapter I'll share some of my menu ideas, but more importantly you'll discover how to find your own way to low-fat eating.

I was in a drugstore the other day, and a doctor and his wife were standing beside a magazine rack looking for a particular magazine. Another doctor came in and recognized them. The wife of the first doctor told the other doctor that they were on the Weight Watcher's Program and had lost weight. The other doctor said he had shed a few pounds also and was happy about it. He then added that he had eaten more lettuce the last two weeks than he had eaten in his entire lifetime. I thought to myself, "How sad! This medical person doesn't understand the secret to energy use in his body."

Friend, you do not have to limit your diet to eating lettuce or being starved. All you need is to educate yourself. You need to learn where the fat is hidden in your diet. That is one thing I hope you understand after you have read this book.

Finding the Hidden Fat

In my constant reading and studying, I have learned from the experts that excessive fat intake is the major contributor to obesity, our number one medical problem. People who are overweight do not intentionally eat too much fat; usually they are unaware of the great amounts of fat in many of the foods they eat.

This lack of information about hidden fat is probably the main reason most people fail to lose weight. They do not realize the fat content in the food they are eating. Once you learn a food is high in fat, you can replace it with another food that is lower in fat.

Changes like this can save you hundreds of fat calories and bring your weight down. A sensible, educated way of eating, coupled with daily exercise, will slim your body, give you energy, and ensure many more productive, healthy days.

I read a report that said the excess fat calories in the American diet aren't just from butter, salad dressings, and ice cream, but they are mainly from high-fat "protein" foods such as meats, fish, poultry, cheese, eggs, and milk.

Have you ever wondered what your daily requirements are for fat, protein, or carbohydrates? Well, I have, and I did some research. Here's what I found out. The calories we get from fat should not exceed 30 percent of our daily calorie intake. Unless you are starving, you will get the required amount of the three essential fatty acids from the protein and carbohydrate foods you are eating.

Lean Foods and Fat Foods

Some people who want to lose weight don't want to fool with calorie counting or knowing the fat content of the food they eat. They say, "Just tell me what to eat and I'll eat it." In this chapter, I will do both. I'll give you some general information regarding fat content in common foods and some low-fat menu ideas.

I hope you will use the fat percentage information to build your own low-fat plan for eating. You can continue to eat many of your favorite foods and still lose weight *if* you find out where the fat is hiding in them and get rid of it.

Robert E. T. Stark, M.D., has written a book titled *Controlling Fat for Life,* as well as a booklet, *The Percent Fat Calories Tables.* This chapter contains information I learned from reading Dr. Stark's books.

The average American diet is over 40 percent fat. We need to bring our fat intake down to where it is only 25 to 30 percent of our total calories. Foods below 30 percent in fat are referred to as "lean foods" and foods over 30 percent fat are considered "fatty foods." The following is a breakdown of percentages.

Below 30%—Lean Foods	Above 30%—Fatty Foods
Trace to 20%—very low fat	30-40%—medium fat
20-30%—low fat	40-60%—high fat
	60-80%—very high fat
	over 80%—extreme fat

Begin to think in terms of "lean foods" and "fat foods." Remember, lean foods consist of foods having a trace of fat to 20 percent (very low fat) and 20 to 30 percent (low fat). The fatty foods (or foods above 30 percent fat) are made up of the following: 30 to 40 percent (medium fat); 40 to 60 percent (high fat); 60 to 80 percent (very high fat); and over 80 percent (extreme fat).

In his booklet, *The Percent Fat Calories Tables,* Dr. Stark breaks down food items into different categories showing the percent of the calories coming from fat.

Fruit: Trace to 5 Percent Fat

These are examples of fruit or complex carbohydrates whose fat content is very low:

apples	bananas
cantaloupe	grapefruit
grapes	honeydew melon
oranges	peaches
pears	strawberries

Most fruit is low in total calories and fat calories. Fruits are an excellent source of food for the low-fat diet.

Vegetables: Trace to Less Than 10 Percent Fat

Vegetables, another form of complex carbohydrates, are a very valuable part of any low-fat, healthy diet. Listed below are some excellent vegetables:

asparagus	lima beans
green beans	beets
broccoli	brussels sprouts
cabbage	carrots
cauliflower	collards
corn	onions
peas	peppers
potatoes	spinach
squash	tomatoes

Meat and Meat Products

The following categories show the percentage of fat in meat and meat products, beginning with the lowest range of calories coming from fat.

20 to 30 percent fat (This is a desirable fat range for you.)

lean hamburger
lamb (leg)
veal (rump, lean)
liver (beef)
turkey (breast)

30 to 40 percent fat

    beef (flank, steak, rib roast, sirloin tip)
    liver (calf)
    corned beef loaf
    ham (lean)
    turkey ham
    turkey pastrami

40 to 60 percent fat

    beef (corned, hamburger—medium fat—
    porterhouse, rib steak, rump, T-bone)
    lamb chop
    pork (Canadian bacon)
    veal cutlet
    lunch meats (chicken roll, sliced ham)

60 to 80 percent fat

    beef (club steak, chuck stew meat)
    lamb (rib chop)
    pork (bacon—medium fat)
    veal (loin chop)
    lunch meats (bologna, corned beef)
    potted meat (canned Spam, Treet)

Over 80 percent fat

    beef (brisket, filet mignon)
    pork (bacon, fat, spare ribs)
    lunch meats (bologna, beef and pork, hot dogs,
    pepperoni)
    canned deviled ham spread, vienna sausages

Choose meats from the two lowest categories. The foods listed in the remaining columns are high-fat content foods.

Soup

Soup is an excellent food but can have varying amounts of fat in it. Listed below is a breakdown showing the percentage of fat in soup.

Zero to 20 percent fat (excellent choice)
    bean
    beef broth
    chicken rice
    tomato rice
    vegetable

20 to 30 percent fat (very good)
    bean with bacon
    beef
    beef and noodle
    chicken noodle
    chicken rice
    clam chowder, Manhattan
    minestrone
    tomato
    vegetable beef

30 to 40 percent fat
    bean with pork
    chicken cream
    onion
    tomato made with milk

40 to 60 percent fat
    asparagus cream
    clam chowder
    New England chowder
    cream of potato
    (Most cream soups come within this category.)

Cheese

These are just a few examples of the many, many types of cheeses. Remember that cheese is a high-fat food, so you want limited amounts of it in your diet.

Zero to 20 percent fat
  low-fat cottage cheese

20 to 40 percent fat
  American low calorie processed
  cottage cheese (creamed, 1/2 cup)
  lite cheeses
  parmesan

60 to 80 percent fat
  American (cheese spread)
  blue
  cheddar
  colby
  cream
  mozzarella (part skim—56 percent fat calories)
  Swiss

Dairy Products

Zero to 20 percent fat
  skim milk
  low-fat yogurt (fruit flavored)

20 to 30 percent fat
  buttermilk
  skim milk yogurt

40 to 60 percent fat
  whole milk
  egg nog
  yogurt (from whole milk)
  ice cream

Over 80 percent fat
   butter
   cream
   whipping cream

Bread, Buns, and Rolls

Zero to 20 percent fat
   bagels
   breads (all kinds—pita, whole wheat, rye, etc.)
   buns
   corn pone
   rolls
   tortillas

20 to 30 percent fat
   rolls (brown and serve)
   pancakes (one medium homemade)

30 to 40 percent fat
   corn sticks
   muffins
   popovers
   waffles
   taco shells

40 to 60 percent fat
   biscuits (homemade)
   corn spoon bread
   croissants
   doughnuts
   french toast

Cereals (Ready-to-Serve)

Zero to 10 percent fat
   All Bran
   Bran Flakes

Cherrios
Grapenuts
oatmeal
Puffed Rice
Shredded Wheat
Special K
Wheaties

Cooked Cereal Served Hot:
cream of wheat
oatmeal
rice
rolled oats
wheat

Cereals are low in fat and are good foods to include in your diet.

Whole-Grain Cereal Products (other than breakfast foods)

Zero to 20 percent fat
corn meal
macaroni
noodles
popcorn
spaghetti
rice

30 to 40 percent fat
spaghetti with cheese and tomato sauce
wheat germ (commercial)

40 to 50 percent fat
macaroni and cheese (baked)
popcorn with oil
spaghetti with Italian-style sauce

Nuts and Seeds

Zero to 20 percent fat
chestnuts

20 to 40 percent fat
soybean nuts

60 to 80 percent fat
cashews
peanuts
sunflower seed kernels
almonds
brazil nuts
pecans
walnuts

Nuts are high in fat. Most fall within the 60-80% fat range.

Robert E. T. Stark, M. D., in his booklet *The Percent Fat Calories Tables,* provides a much more comprehensive breakdown of the percent of calories coming from fat. Entire sections are devoted to fish and seafood, poultry and game, and beef cuts.

Dr. Stark also breaks down the percentage of fat for crackers, cookies, appetizers and snacks, sweets, candies, desserts, fats and oils, and even fast-foods. If you haven't ordered this little booklet, please do so immediately. It will really teach you how to zero in on the fat in your diet.

Where Does Fat Fit In?

In his book, *Controlling Fat for Life,* Dr. Stark tells us that back in the 1950s, the nutritional authorities classified our foods into four basic food groups:

1 *Meat, fish, and poultry*—Mainly protein foods with calories coming from protein and fat.

2. *Fruits and vegetables*—These are carbohydrate foods with calories from carbohydrates and a few from protein and fat.

3. *Breads, cereals, and starchy vegetables*—These are carbohydrate foods with calories from carbohydrates and some from protein and fat.

4. *Dairy products*—These are fat foods such as milk, butter, and cheese. Calories mainly come from fat but some come from carbohydrate and protein.

At one time it was easy to classify food into each of these food groups, or so we thought. Today it is not so simple. You might assume chicken comes under the food group of meat, fish, and poultry. But when it is fried in high-fat oil, this high-protein food ends up with over twice as many calories from fat as from protein. Fried chicken, as prepared in most fast-food restaurants, can no longer be considered a protein food but rather a fat food.

Milk is a dairy product with half its calories coming from fat. Skim milk, however, is primarily a protein-carbohydrate food with only 2 percent of its calories from fat. Skim milk and cottage cheese made from skim milk are practically devoid of fat and should be considered a high-protein food.

Potatoes and onions are vegetables with very few fat calories. When fried, these vegetables take on a new flavor and a lot of fat calories. The fat-calorie content of these foods is increased 40 times when they are fried. With onion rings, the fat calories are 80 percent of the total. This moves these two vegetables from the classification of vegetables to a high-fat food classfication with most calories coming from fat and few from carbohydrates.

The calories in our food and drink come from carbohydrates, fat, and protein. In each food group, one of the three food sources of calories is dominant. For example, in fruits and vegetables, we think of carbohydrates as being the main food source. In nuts and cheese, we think of fat as being the dominant food source, and we think of protein as being the dominant food source in lean meat, poultry, and fish. Whenever food is processed or when it has a high fat content, the major source of its calories will be fat.

Carbohydrates are found mainly in fruits and vegetables and in breads, cereals and starchy vegetables. Fat calories come mainly from meat, fish, poultry and dairy products. In dairy products, fats are the chief source of calories.

Determining Percentage of Fat

I am often asked, "Beverly, how do I know if a food has too much fat just from reading the label?"

In order to find the percentage of fat in food, multiply the number of fat grams by 9. This will give you the total fat calories. Then this number must be divided by the total calories. If the answer you get is over 30 percent, then the food is a fat food.

You multiply the fat grams by 9 because 9 is the number of calories in a gram of fat. Total calories are to be divided into total fat grams. This shows you the number of calories from fat compared to the total calories in food.

For example, a waffle has 7 grams of fat. Multiply 7 by 9 and you get 63 fat calories. The total calories in the waffle is 140, so divide the 63 fat calories by the 140 total calories and the answer is 45 percent. This is over 30 percent fat even before you add the butter or syrup, so this would be one food to avoid.

Any food that has 50 percent of its calories from fat is a fat food. Cheddar cheese is a fat food because over 50 percent of its calories come from fat. Some foods, like lunch meats, are thought to be protein, but 60 to 80 percent of their calories come from fat.

Give Up Dessert?

Sugar foods like doughnuts, chocolate candy bars, and cookies have more fat calories than sugar calories so they are a fat food. Since sugar is a simple carbohydrate, some people think of sugar foods as only carbohydrates; but the large number of calories make them mainly a fat food.

Candies become fatty foods when either chocolate or nuts or both are added. In other words, candies have more calories from fat than from sugar. Read all labels to check the content of protein, fat, and calories. Start training yourself in nutrition this way.

Some desserts are low in fat and have a high-carbohydrate content. Examples would be angel food cake, sponge cake, D-Zerta, jellos, ices, sherbets, and tapioca. Some desserts are low-fat, but have large amounts of calories due to high-sugar content. Even though they are low in fat, you will want to avoid them if you want to lose weight.

Desserts containing chocolate will have a high-fat content because chocolate is a high fat-caloric food. Here are some true fat desserts: pies, ice cream, cakes, turnovers, Danish pastries, brownies, and cream puffs.

The person interested in weight loss will want to eat complex carbohydrates like fruits, vegetables, and whole grains. These foods nourish the body without adding fat. You could say that all carbohydrates are not created equal— the complex ones do more for you!

The 100 percent fat foods are butter, margarine, and oils that are used mainly in cooking and for flavoring. These foods are high in fat, but any food over 40 percent in fat content will cause people to put on weight. Every day we eat good, nutritious foods—like nuts and cheeses—without recognizing their fat content. These are good foods, but if you are trying to reduce, see them as high-fat foods!

Here are some specific food items and their fat percentages:

> nuts and seeds—60-80% fat
> cheese—60-80% (except skim milk, low-fat variety)

soups can be from 20% up to 80% depending on
fat content
vegetables and fruits—0-under 20% fat (usually
low)
eggs—60-80% (leave out yolk and they are low
fat)
cereals—0-20% fat
crackers—can be anywhere from 20 to 60% fat
cookies—40-60% fat
candies—40-60% fat
fats and oils—100% fat
butter—100% fat
salad dressings—80% fat
sauces and gravies—80% fat
fast-food—up to 80% fat
biscuit—60% fat

Remember, we want our diet 30 percent fat or lower in
order to lose weight or be healthy. Foods that are below 30
percent are low-fat foods. As fat calorie percentages increase
above 30 percent, the degree of fatness in you and your diet
increases.

Finding The Hidden Fat

There are a couple of common foods I want you to watch
out for. Peanut butter falls in the range of 60 to 80 percent
fat calories, and tartar sauce is 95 percent fat calories. I knew
these two were high in fat, but I never imagined they were
that high.

I was reviewing a report on fast-food restaurants. Their
burgers, chicken and fish sandwiches all fall within the 50
percent fat calorie range. These are truly fat foods and meals.

We need to recognize fat foods and see if there are ways
we can change our diet to lower our daily fat intake. An
example of fat reduction might be with eggs. Eggs are in the

60 to 80 percent fat calorie range. If, however, you scramble the whites only, your fat intake will be reduced to the 0 to 20 percent range.

One viewer wrote that when she scrambled eggs for her family, she would use three eggs but only one yolk—the other two yolks she discarded.

A bagel or other such breads are low in fat, falling in the range of 0-20 percent fat calories. But a homemade biscuit is in the 40-60 percent fat calorie category. The same is true with pancakes. In addition to the pancake being a high-fat food, the butter and syrup you add to it increases fat content even more. If you had a wholesome cereal with sliced banana and skim milk, you would have had a very low-fat breakfast with lots of energy for the day.

Planning the Low-Fat Menu

I like foods that are easy to prepare. I like simple eating. I know few people who have time to prepare six-course dinners from scratch. I am one of those people who do not enjoy spending a lot of time at the kitchen stove.

At breakfast, I am especially in a hurry. I exercise and have devotions in the morning. I am not able to plan breakfasts that require much preparation time. Yet knowing that breakfast is the most important meal of the day, I must be careful to find a nutritious and quick way of eating for myself and my family.

The first breakfast I am about to describe is my favorite, and it is highly nutritious while being low in fat. You cannot go wrong with a low-sugar, high-fiber cereal/fruit combination.

Eating With Beverly

Following are two, whole-day menus that provide an example of what I eat. I urge you to use the previous information along with ideas from my sample menus to make up your own low-fat menus. You'll be glad you did.

Day One Menu

Breakfast: Oatmeal (cooks in one minute)
             Combine it with shredded wheat/raisin
             bite size biscuits
             Top with sliced banana and skim milk.

Lunch: Baked potato with chili
             Top with part-skim milk cheese
             Salad (lettuce, cucumbers, tomatoes)
             Low-fat salad dressing
             Pita Bread
             Skim Milk
             Pear for dessert

Dinner: Plate of pasta with tomato sauce
             Topped with part-skim mozzarella cheese
             Rye bread
             Lettuce salad with cottage cheese
             Apple for dessert

Bedtime   Bite-Size Shredded Wheat with
Snack: fruit inside the biscuit
             A few grapes

I drink lots of water throughout the day. I run three miles first thing in the morning on an empty stomach. I exercise at 6:00 a.m. with ankle and wrist weights. So I am really ready for breakfast at 6:30 a.m. I have found this breakfast to be completely satisfying.

Day Two Menu

Breakfast: Scrambled egg (scrambled in Pam spray)
Heated pita bread
Fresh strawberries
Skim milk

Lunch: Progresso soup with cooked broccoli,
onions, and potatoes (I always add my
own steamed vegetables to canned
soup to lower the sodium content.)
Pita bread with salmon (I use canned
salmon. This sandwich will consist of
lettuce and salmon on pita bread.)
Skim milk
Banana for dessert

Dinner: Chicken breast (baked in oven in oven
bag with skin removed)
Rice
Peas
Carrots
Fresh spinach salad with low-fat dressing
Grapes and fresh strawberries for dessert
Whole wheat bread
Skim milk

Bedtime
Snack: Popcorn (popped in microwave with no
salt or oil)

Day Three Menu

Breakfast: Hot Cereal (I like oatmeal.)
Banana
Warm pita bread
Skim milk for cereal
Orange

Lunch: Collards (or other greens high in
            nutrition)
            Boiled potatoes
            Lima beans
            Corn
            Corn bread*
            Cantaloupe and strawberries for dessert
            (*See no-oil recipe for corn bread
            below.)

Dinner: Baked fish
            Broccoli
            Rice
            Whole wheat bread
            Fruit for dessert

As you can see, I eat simple foods. Make your own selection from the lists I've provided and by using Dr. Stark's booklet. Your diet should be made up of 55-60% complex carbohydrates. These include fruits, vegetables, and whole grains. Look for the foods that are the lowest in fat. Put your own combinations together. This is so much better than being told what to eat. Train yourself *not* to eat sweets and fried foods. Develop a taste for fruits for dessert, and you will always want them. You can learn to love the low-fat way of eating. I promise.

No-Oil Corn Bread Recipe

Heat oven to 450 degrees. Spray skillet with Pam or any non-stick vegetable spray. Place skillet in oven to get it hot. Remove hot skillet, and pour prepared corn bread mixture into it. Here's how to mix it:
    2 Cups self-rising corn meal
    1 Egg   Skim milk
Add skim milk until mixture is smooth enough for pouring
Pour into hot skillet and bake 25 minutes at 400 degrees.

————16————
Changes You Can
Live With

Many families still eat fried foods, especially meats like chicken, fish, and hamburgers. Even though these foods are very good for you, too many times they have hidden fat in them because of the way they are prepared. With simple changes in ingredients, seasonings, and preparation techniques, you can still eat many of your favorite foods and maintain a low-fat diet.

Fats contain the highest number of calories per gram. Consider that a single gram of butter—a minute quantity about the size of one small pea—contains 7.2 calories. A gram of corn, olive, or peanut oil supplies a staggering 8.9 calories. That's 40 to 50 calories in one teaspoon!

These figures help explain why fats contribute such a high percentage of calories—around 40 percent—to the American diet. According to the Congressional commission on nutrition, fats have now replaced sugar as dietary enemy number one. Fats, especially saturated fats found in meat and dairy products, raise the blood cholesterol level. Fatty foods are linked to heart disease and arteriosclerosis.

You honestly may not see where you have any obvious fats in your diet. That's because most of the fat is hidden in the food itself—either naturally or through preparation. For example, if you put a regular dressing on your salad, as much as 90 percent of the calories in that salad might come from fat. You can eat salad every meal and still gain weight—depending on your dressings and how much cheese and other high-fat foods are added.

Substituting Low-Fat Foods

Some dieters cringe at the thought of totally eliminating certain foods from their diets. You will want to avoid high-fat foods like red meat, whole milk and whole-milk products such as ice cream, whole-milk cheese, and sour cream. But does that mean you can never enjoy food again?

No! Many of these foods can be replaced by other foods that are lower in fat and better for you. Skim milk has more calcium and just a fraction of the fat that whole milk contains. Many people don't feel they're sacrificing by making the switch.

Ice milk or sherbet can satisfy your taste for something sweet without overloading your fat cells like rich desserts or fattening ice creams. Substituting low-fat yogurt for sour cream can save you as much as 349 calories per cup.

What about the "spreadable inedibles" like butter and mayonnaise? Switch to margarine, which is better for you. Tub margarines are generally softer and less saturated than stick margarines. Diet brands are even better. Substitute mustard, ketchup, or relish for mayonnaise on sandwiches. Add yogurt to mayonnaise to cut the fat content or buy a low-fat brand from the dietetic section of your grocery store.

Cheese may be the most difficult food to cut from your diet. The average American eats 26 pounds of it per year. While being a good source of minerals and vitamins, cheese calories are 65 to 75 percent fat. A typical one-ounce serving or slice of cheese contains almost the same amount of fat as two pats of butter. Cheese fat is saturated fat that raises blood cholesterol and increases the risk of heart disease.

Avoid all high-fat cheeses. Instead use low-fat cottage cheese or part-skim ricotta cheese (this can replace cream cheese in a recipe or spread).

At the Grocery Store

Your resolve to start a low-fat diet will be tested as you wheel your grocery cart through the aisles of chips, dip, snack food, baked goods, and desserts. How can you ensure success when you emerge from the check-out line?

First, write out a grocery list and stick to it. If you plan your meals ahead of time, you'll be less tempted to run out at the last minute and buy something unhealthy. Always have low-fat food in stock.

Second, read labels to check the fat content of foods. Multiply fat grams by nine and divide that by the total number of calories to find the percentage of fat in foods. Labels must list the most prominent ingredients by weight in descending order. Obviously, if the first ingredient is fat, oil, sugar, or salt, you'll want to leave it on the shelf.

Third, cut your fat content by shopping wisely. If you don't buy it, you can't eat it.

Using common sense in shopping can cut calories and fat from your diet. Select canned fruits that are packed in their own juices, not sweet syrups. Water-packed tuna has 13 fat calories compared to 339 fat calories in oil-packed varieties. Frozen vegetables are great, but avoid the ones that come with butter or cheese sauces.

What about selecting meats? How do you know what has the least fat content? "Good" has the least fat; "choice" has more; and "prime" has the most. Foods that count as little else but fat are bologna, hotdogs, sausage, and salami. Baked or smoked turkey, baked or boiled ham or roast beef are much lower in fat and much better for you.

Preparation Tips

Now that you've gotten the groceries home, how do you prepare low-fat meals? If you've selected low-fat foods, you don't want to ruin all your planning with poor preparation.

How you prepare your food also affects the nutritional value of your diet. For example, a salad that was prepared two or three days ago has lost most of its nutritional value. Overcooking also destroys nutrients.

Go for variety in the food choices on your diet. For example, adding broccoli to your salad contributes vitamin A. The more variety you have the better your chances of getting all the vitamins and minerals you require.

Frying is a real mistake for the dieter. You can fry a low-fat cup of potatoes and add as much as 217 fat calories. Twice the fat lies in fried chicken as opposed to roasted chicken. You can double the calories in a serving of pasta by adding one tablespoon of butter or margarine.

You can decrease the oil or shortening in most recipes by as much as one-third to one-half the amount called for without damaging flavor. Just be sure to compensate for the missing liquid by adding low-fat milk or any other low-fat liquid that would be appropriate. When possible use skim milk since it has no fat grams in eight ounces as compared to 9 grams of fat in the same amount of whole milk.

What about eggs? You may want to keep egg substitutes on hand because of their lower fat and cholesterol. Egg substitutes allow you to enjoy omelets and french toast without the dangers of real egg yolks. They usually are high in sodium, however.

What About Meats?

How do you prepare meats without causing their fat content to skyrocket? Trim all visible fat from any meats you eat. Remove chicken skins as the first stage in preparation. Remember a little goes a long way when it comes to fat.

Some key factors for fat control in your daily preparation of meats include:

1. Instead of frying, sautee meats and vegetables in a nonstick pan sprayed lightly with vegetable spray.
2. Stir-fry meats and vegetables in 1 to 2 teaspoons of oil. (Have some chicken broth handy to finish the job.)
3. Steam vegetables, fish, and chicken with water or chicken broth.
4. Broil meats on drip racks in oven. (Never baste with fat drippings. Baste with chicken broth, beef broth or vegetable juices.)
5. Add a few ice-cubes to meat drippings to harden the fat so you can skim it off before making gravy. The fat will cling to the ice cubes.
6. Chill canned meats, broths, and stews before opening the can so you can skim off the hardened fat.

Serve smaller portions of meats than you have normally been doing. We eat much more meat than we need. Better yet, make meat part of a casserole or stir fry chunks of meat in with vegetables and olive oil. Meat cut in strips will satisfy the meat lover by giving him the impression he is eating a lot more than he really is.

What's in a Name?

Pure vegetable oil. Sounds healthy, doesn't it? No animal fat means it must be good. Not necessarily. Some pure vegetable oil is more saturated than beef tallow, which is used in the making of soap and candles. Beef tallow is 50 percent saturated fat—the worst kind of fat.

Coconut oil, in which many snack foods are cooked, is 86 percent saturated fat! Those delicious snacks get much of their flavor and crunch from fatty oils such as coconut oil. Food manufacturers like to use palm and coconut oils because they are cheaper and help preserve the food. Read the labels and see what kind of oils are being used in your favorite foods.

One of the major ingredients to look for is "hydrogenated oils," especially palm and coconut oils. Hydrogenation is a process that hardens or hydrogenates an unsaturated oil, making it saturated. Stick margarine is an example of corn oil that has been hydrogenated to hold its shape. Hydrogenated oils are common in crackers, bakery products, convenience foods, and non-dairy creamers.

Poly, Mono, and Un

All oils provide vitamin E. Wheat-germ, safflower, cotton-seed, corn, and almond oils also boast very high amounts of vitamin K. Each molecule of oil is composed of three fatty acids linked to each other by a small bridging unit called glycerol. The size of the fatty acid molecule and its average number of double bonds, or its degree of unsaturation, determine how it affects your health.

If there is only one double bond, a fatty acid is called *monounsaturated.* If there are more, it is called *polyunsaturated.* One polyunsaturate, linoleic acid, must be present in the diet because the body needs it but cannot make it on its own. Good sources of linoleic acid are corn, cotton-seed, safflower, soybean, and sunflower oils. One tablespoon of any one of these oils meets your body's daily needs for linoleic acid.

Once that one tablespoon is in your body, no one seems sure how much more fatty acids are needed by the body. Most experts do agree, however, that the fat intake for adults must be kept low for the health of the heart and the colon.

Since no vegetable oil contains cholesterol, what you must pay attention to is saturated fat in coconut oil, palm oil, and pure butter. A reasonable diet should include about half its fatty acid in monounsaturates, one-third as saturates, and the remaining sixth as polyunsaturates. The following table clearly defines the fat percentages in most common oils. You can see from this table why I choose to use safflower oil.

Oil	Saturated %	Unsaturated %	
		Poly	Mono
Coconut	92	6	2
Corn	13	25	62
Olive	14	77	9
Palm	53	38	9
Peanut	18	48	34
Safflower	9	13	78
Sesame	14	42	44
Soybean	15	25	60
Sunflower	11	21	68
Butter	68	28	4
Lard	41	43	16
Soft Margarine	19	53	28
Shortening	25	68	7

Remember, oils high in saturated fats are the least desirable because they promote elevation of blood cholesterol.

What About Seasonings?

People often tell me they season their vegetables with salt pork. Salt pork is 98 percent fat. When added to green beans or other vegetables, salt pork turns a low-fat food into a high-fat food. Those vegetables skyrocket from a zero to 10 percent fat range to 60 to 80 percent. The fat hidden in your green beans will soon be in your fat cells. Changes in seasonings can mean the difference between a lean or a fat food.

The use of non-stick pans or sprays is highly beneficial in cutting fat. The food may not be quite as tasty as that prepared with butter, but you can spice it up with herbs, broths, or olive oil. In seasoning vegetables, use herbs and spices or a harmless oil like oriental sesame oil instead of fatback meat or heavy oils.

Can Salt Make You Fat?

Salt is truly dangerous and is directly linked to high blood pressure. Eating less salt usually results in weight loss and reduced hypertension. Salt is known to cause weight swings and bloating, which lead to high blood pressure.

Can salt make you fat? Since salt causes the body's tissues to retain water, a low-salt diet has long been standard practice for anyone wanting to reduce. We thought the weight loss was due to water loss, but the *British Medical Journal* reports that salt affects the body's absorption of food as well.

After eating, the body's blood sugar level rises in response to the amount and type of food we eat. Researchers gave unsalted food to a study group and the blood sugar levels increased. When salt was added to the meals, however, the blood sugar levels increased more.

Salt either enhanced digestion so that more sugar was released from the food or it stimulated the intestines to absorb sugar more efficiently. The evidence seems to say that adding salt to a meal increases the number of calories absorbed by the body.

Salt—Who Needs It?

The salt lover's greatest nightmare is a meal without salt. People accustomed to the salty flavor fear the food will have no taste. Actually just the opposite is true. Reducing salt brings out the natural flavors in food.

The salt addict is like any other addict. He can't just drop salt cold turkey. Gradually decreasing your salt intake may be easier unless you have high blood pressure and your doctor has ordered you to quit immediately. Your taste buds will adjust and eventually prefer a less salty or even no-salt taste.

Once you kick the salt habit, you are also on your way to kicking the junk food habit. As you grow accustomed to less salt, the salty nuts, chips, and sandwich meats associated with snack foods will become entirely too salty for your taste. If you must buy processed foods, choose the low-salt items as much as possible. If you must snack, use low-salt snacks.

But let's face it. Some foods are bland, even blah without salt. So what can you do with them? Try seasoning your food with herbs, spices, garlic, onions, peppers, vinegars, lemons, limes, and curry.

What About Salt Substitutes?

Beware of salt substitutes. If the label says it contains potassium chloride, don't use it without first talking with your doctor. Don't expect salt substitutes to take the place of salt and do not use them as freely as you would salt.

Most salt substitutes contain a warning label that says they are not to be used under certain circumstances or without the advice of a doctor. Because they are so readily available on the grocery shelf, most people do not heed the warning, if they read it at all.

The Journal of the *American Medical Association* warns that potassium, which replaces sodium in salt substitutes, can be toxic in large quantities. This substance can accumulate in the blood and tissues, causing muscle weakness and heart disturbances. The chances of this happening increase when certain medications are being taken.

The person who switches to a low-fat, low-salt diet need not fear that mealtimes will be boring, bland, and tasteless for the rest of her life. She can continue to eat many of the same foods she has always enjoyed by modifying the way they are prepared, seasoned, and served.

Cutting the Fat from Your Diet

Dieters must derive pleasure from the food they eat. The quantity of filling carbohydrates one can eat conquers any feeling of deprivation. Don't be afraid to cut the fat and fill up on complex carbohydrates.

That's what I do. For example, I sometimes have a high-fiber cereal with banana for breakfast; maybe soup for lunch with lots of my own steamed or microwaved vegetables added so there will be lots of fiber and less salt. I eat the soup with pita bread and top it off with an apple for dessert. For dinner I'll have spaghetti (again high fiber) with just a little sauce, a large salad with low-fat dressing, and a large pear for dessert.

On a diet like this, you're never hungry so you won't be tempted to raid the refrigerator later. Be sure to have a glass of skim milk with your lunch and dinner in order to get the calcium you need. This low-fat way of eating is guaranteed to keep you satisfied.

Americans need to cut their fat intake by one-half. If you give up one-half of your fat intake and replace it with starches, it would be possible to lose as much as one pound a week just from this action alone.

By replacing fats such as butter and oil with carbohydrates like bread, potatoes, pastas, and rice, many dieters have found they feel more satisfied. By eating in moderation and restricting your fats, you are likely to achieve the kind of remarkable weight loss that usually results only from the most strict low-calorie diet.

17

You Can Enjoy Exercising

I can still remember how difficult it was for me to exercise with my allergy-sick body, congested chest, flabby muscles, excess fat, and nicotine-addicted body. In the beginning exercise seemed like torture. My muscles ached for over a week. After exercising, breathing deeply, and drinking lots of water for my first week, I prayed I would live.

What a "jolt" for my body! By the end of the second week I was beginning to experience more energy, less pain, and general loosening of my clothes. Several weeks into my program I was telling myself, "Don't miss a single session, Beverly. Don't quit! It would be so easy to fall back into your old ways."

I really believe fear of quitting kept me faithful as I progressed through those first few weeks of exercise. Now I can thank God for keeping me faithful over the twenty years I have exercised regularly.

If you have never been physically fit, experience it now so you can have one more thing to praise God for. Never in my youth did I enjoy the health and energy that I now experience at age forty-seven. This physical fitness plan God has for us is so exciting.

Remember, our bodies belong to God—we've been bought with a price and we are not our own. (See 1 Corinthians 6:19,20). God wants our bodies strong and healthy to do His work. God doesn't want spiritual wimps!

Making the Investment

The Lord has made our bodies in such a way that often we can make ourselves well if we are willing to work at exercise and diet. Most people know exercise is good for them, they just have a hard time working it into the daily routine they have followed for years.

It takes really "wanting to" to do anything worthwhile, including exercise. We find time for what we want to do, don't we? If people could just realize that exercise is not torture, that it can even be fun, and that the results are worth every drop of sweat and every inconvenience, they would be more willing to commit to it on a regular basis.

Sadly, most people live and die and never experience the joy of a physically fit body. I have often thought to myself, "If only they could experience a physically fit, healthy body for a month, I know most people would never stop eating right and exercising once they had begun."

I prefer to look at exercise as an investment in my health and well-being. To feel fit spiritually and physically, I jog 21 miles per week, do floor exercises each day, eat a low-fat diet, and have daily prayer and Bible reading.

I don't count my housework or work in the yard as exercise. My exercise is my planned program and that should be yours, too. If you garden or mow the grass, fine, but you still need to have a planned exercise time each day—either thirty minutes of walking or indoor exercises.

Exercise should become just as much a part of your life as brushing your teeth. Pick an activity you enjoy so you won't view exercise as punishment for past gastronomic sins. You may enjoy some of the same activities you enjoyed as a child, such as hiking, biking, and swimming. Mark out time in your schedule for exercise and stick to it. Take time to give yourself the gift of exercise.

Work or Play?

Many beginners make the mistake of trying to exercise too much, too soon, and too fast. Going at the exercise game too hard and too fast causes people to quit. You cannot stretch as thoroughly if you exercise too fast. Many of my exercises are based on ballet, which allows for a slower pace and more stretching.

Many people drop out because they choose a form of exercise that cannot be enjoyed. Exercise should fit in with your way of life and who you are. You should look forward to those thirty minutes of activity each day. Choose exercises that will not totally disrupt your life and schedule. Exercise should be enjoyed, not endured.

If you hate exercise, you probably see it as work instead of fun. Just stop and watch children at play. They're exercising— but they're having a great time doing it. That's because all they know is that they're having fun. It hasn't occurred to them that skipping rope or playing tag is exercise.

Most work used to be exercise, but riding mowers and automatic machines of every sort changed all that. Doing normal everyday chores does not provide us with nearly the same benefits that our grandparents derived from comparable tasks.

We still continue to associate exercise with work. But you can do something about that. Find a method of exercise that is so enjoyable that exercising becomes secondary to the fact that you're having fun! Exercise should be like play— something you enjoy and look forward to each day.

Some people drop out of exercise because they don't exercise carefully or properly and therefore derive little benefit. What's my approach to exercise? I believe in giving it my best and doing it right. Dress for your exercise session in a snappy, comfortable outfit suitable for what you are doing. Give your exercise time priority and a place of respect in your life. Making that commitment and then sticking with it will give your mind and body a lift.

Benefits of Exercise

Our bodies seem to have a built-in ability to balance the calories we consume with the calories we use. But without exercise, this mechanism does not work properly. The less active we are, the more pounds we pile on. This explains why, when you eat the same amounts of food at age forty as you did at twenty, you find yourself ten to fifteen pounds heavier unless you have exercised regularly. Inactivity takes its toll.

Some people never have a problem with weight until an accident or illness forces them into a period of inactivity and then—wham—before they know it they're ten or twenty pounds overweight. When you are less active than you were created to be (and the American way is still largely an inactive way), your metabolism goes awry and you begin to lose the battle of the bulge.

As you exercise you lay down more muscle. Most diets fail to keep weight off because they result in a loss of lean muscle mass as well as fat. Whenever you lose weight without exercise, you lose lean muscle mass and very little fat. This slows your metabolism. If you keep this up for a long time, you will end up fatter than when you began to diet. Scientists tell us a diet without exercise can cut your metabolism by as much as 30 percent.

Speeding Up Your Metabolism

Latest research shows that many obese people eat no more than normal-weight people. Their slower metabolisms, however, do not burn fat as efficiently as their leaner counterparts.

One study suggests that one way to speed up a sluggish metabolism is to eat four meals each day. To aid in the digestive process of calorie burning, follow at least two of the meals with a brisk, twenty-minute walk. This can increase the amount of calories burned by as much as 50 percent.

For example, if your natural metabolism normally burns 100 calories during digestion, a brisk walk would increase that amount to 150 calories burned. In a year, you could burn off an extra ten pounds.

If your skinny neighbor can enjoy pie for dessert and never gain a pound, and you can gain ten pounds just by looking at it, her metabolism probably burns off excess calories better than yours. She may be taking a walk after meals. The more calories burned, the less fat stored.

Exercise boosts your metabolism. If you exercise fifteen minutes after eating a meal, you increase the calorie-burning ability of your body. Exercise causes your body to "roast calories." Instead of storing the calories after you eat, you can burn them. You can see how important it is to take a walk or do some mild form of exercise after eating instead of sitting down to read a book.

If you really want to burn calories, add some aerobic exercise at least three times a week to your schedule. You can burn calories for as long as twenty-four hours after a good workout of thirty to forty-five minutes. At the same time you are increasing muscle mass and reducing fat stores.

Larger muscles need more calories to function. For each pound of muscle added to your body, an additional 50 to 100 calories a day are burned in order for the muscles to function. The more muscle you have the more efficient your metabolism because muscle tissue is more active than fat tissue.

Exercise and Your Ideal Weight

Exercise is a good way to lower your set point weight. Your normal body weight is similar to water—it seeks its own level. Your set point is the weight you maintain when you are making no special effort to gain or lose.

If your weight drops below your set point, your body automatically begins a struggle to climb back up to that set point. A starvation signal to the brain triggers defense systems that actually cause diet after diet to fail.

The only way to win the set point battle is to lower your normal weight to a lower level through exercise. You can actually reset your set point weight to a lower level.

When you tell someone that it takes sixteen hours of walking to lose one pound, they want to give up on exercise before they begin. But exercise does far more than burn a few on-the-spot calories for you. Exercise raises your metabolism and speeds up your system so that your body continues to burn calories for several hours after you stop exercising.

For example, if you exercise thirty minutes twice a day—once in the morning and once in the evening—you are burning extra calories all day, even as you sleep. Even if you know you have a slow metabolism, you can permanently speed it up with exercise.

Replacing Fat Tissue

Research has shown that exercising within two to three hours after you've eaten gives you good results. More calories seem to be burned on a full stomach than on an empty one. The extra body heat produced during exercise makes this possible.

When you exercise is important but not as important as just exercising. I believe exercising after a meal is greatly beneficial. Since eating itself raises the metabolic rate, if you do a mild form of exercise after eating, it stands to reason that the metabolic rate would increase even more. Instead of sitting right down after a meal, walk around the block a few times.

This bears repeating—regular exercise replaces fat tissue with lean muscle mass. Since lean tissue uses more calories to sustain itself than fat, the more lean tissue you build up, the easier it becomes to burn calories.

Lean tissue takes up less space than fat. Even if you don't see an immediate decrease in pounds after starting an exercise program, you'll look thinner because you'll be taking up less space. When the mirror says you look fit and trim, who cares what the scales say?

What Have You Got to Lose?

Did you know that you can go from being a big, fat person to being a little, fat person? You may lose weight, but your tissue remains fat. Only when exercise is included in a weight-loss program can a person reduce fat tissue to lean muscle mass.

If you have ever seen an arm that has been in a cast for three months, that arm is much smaller than the healthy arm. This is because the muscle mass on the broken arm wasted away from disuse while in the cast. As you look at the loose, flabby skin on the broken arm and compare it to the healthy arm, you can get a picture of just how important exercise is.

Between the ages of twenty-five and fifty-five, a person who does not exercise loses fifteen pounds of lean muscle mass. This loss occurs throughout the body and in its place comes fifteen pounds of fat. You may weigh the same at age fifty-five as you did at eighteen, but if you have not exercised your measurements will not be the same. You might find that you are very small in the shoulders and larger in the hips and thighs. For example, you might wear a size five top and a size ten bottom.

In addition to replacing fifteen pounds of muscle with fifteen pounds of fat, the average person will gain ten pounds of body fat every decade. Between age twenty-five and fifty-five, the average person gains thirty pounds of fat due to lack of exercise. By age fifty-five, a person who does not exercise can have forty-five additional pounds of fat on him.

Muscle mass can be rebuilt through exercise. Even if you are sixty-five today and have never exercised, if you start walking about thirty minutes a day and begin working with me, your body will immediately begin to develop lean muscle mass. Lean muscles are actually the "engines" of the body that burn calories. Fat just goes along for the ride. You are never too old to start building lean muscle mass and increasing metabolism. Daily exercise will do this for you—regardless of your age.

What You Don't Want to Lose

When you go on a crash diet, the first pounds you lose are fluid. This is a temporary loss at best. After fluid, the next thing you begin losing is protein and muscle tissue. You don't want this to happen because muscle tissue is needed for a good body shape. The sudden loss of muscle protein can make you too tired to exercise. Loss of muscle tissue leads to a quick re-gain of weight once the diet ends.

You have to be on a crash diet several weeks before you start burning up stored fat. The same diet that let you quickly shed five pounds of fluid will only take off one pound of fat during the next week or two. This is where people become discouraged and quit.

So how can you begin to lose fat immediately? The only way is through exercise. Only exercise allows you to keep your lean muscle and even increase it while burning fat for energy. No diet will do this for you. Losing weight through dieting alone will eat away at your lean muscle tissue and can even become life-threatening. If an extremely low-calorie diet continues, the loss of muscle tissue extends to every organ of your body including the heart.

Slow and Steady

Exercise may seem slow and hard next to some miracle diet powder, but the losses you gain through exercise are permanent. You will end up smaller and firmer not smaller and still fat. A slow loss is a more lasting loss.

A recent study in obesity revealed some interesting results. A group of obese adults who had dieted repeatedly without success were told to forget dieting, eat normally, and take a thirty-minute walk five times a week. Eleven people stuck with this exercise program for a year and a half. How did they fare by disregarding diet and concentrating on exercise? These walkers experienced an *average* weight loss of twenty-two pounds. And their successful weight loss is continuing.

Just remember—newly thin people do not burn calories as fast as those who have always been thin. Their metabolism is much slower. Former "overweights" can pile on an extra five pounds a year just by eating a "normal" diet of 1,900 calories a day unless they find additional ways to burn calories through exercise. A regular, mild exercise has been found to be the kind people will stick with the most—like walking.

Studies have shown that those who chose a strenuous exercise such as dance aerobics could not do it fast enough and long enough to burn many calories. But those who walked regularly could burn as many as 340 additional calories a day.

I know you've heard this before, and you will probably hear it again, but the best formula for weight loss is a low-fat, high-complex carbohydrate diet and regular exercise. That dynamite combination is the key to a smaller, firmer, leaner you.

Additional Benefits of Exercise

Exercise reduces the absorption of calories. When you are active, food passes through your intestinal tract much faster and fewer calories are absorbed. The average person digests a meal in twenty-four hours. In obese people whose inactivity has caused weakened muscles, digestion can take as long as forty-eight hours. An athlete's digestive process may only take four to six hours. The longer food remains in your intestines, the greater the risk of intestinal disorders and even bowel cancer.

Increasing exercise is more important than cutting back on food. Study after study has shown that those who eat a fiber-rich, low-fat diet combined with regular exercise lose much more fat than those who just try to lose with some fad diet or pill.

In a study of exercisers versus non-exercisers that involved an 18-pound weight loss, 11 pounds of fat and 7 pounds of lean muscle mass were lost by the non-exercisers. The exercisers lost 23 pounds of fat and gained 4 pounds of lean muscle mass. In addition to losing weight, the exercisers boosted their metabolism.

Muscle contains a large number of capillaries, which are tiny vessels that transport oxygen-rich blood throughout your body. This blood is used by your body to produce the energy necessary for muscular contractions. Fat does not have to work, so it has no capillary system.

What is the secret to making your body burn calories even as you rest? Increase the size of your muscles. Larger muscles need more calories to function. If you add one pound of muscle to your body, research tells us that your body will then require an additional 50 to 100 calories a day to function. If you begin to exercise and do not add any calories to your diet, you will be dipping into your fat cells for energy to burn. You will lose weight.

A Natural "High"

Exercise is a natural relaxant and gives you a feeling of well-being. If you are relaxed and feel good about yourself, chances are you will not be tempted to binge on food in order to find comfort. The euphoria or well-being one feels after exercise is triggered by hormones produced in the brain called endorphins. The effect of this "natural Valium" is why some people become "addicted" to jogging or other exercise.

Other studies have shown that people who exercise regularly have an improved ability to make quick decisions. One study determined that people who are physically fit are 60 percent more adept at making complex decisions than those who do not exercise regularly. That's not to say that physical fitness improves a person's intellect, it just helps him make the most of what he has.

Lack of exercise can leave you too tired to work or exercise. Studies show that people who complain of being tired all the time are much less fit than those who don't complain. In tests, these people did poorly on the treadmill. Two years later they were tested again, and those who had begun regular exercise programs showed improved performance on the treadmill.

The important thing is to begin—do what little bit of exercising you can. Maybe all you can do at first is walk around the block. You don't have to enter a marathon. Just a little bit of exercise will increase your energy and improve your outlook on life.

Defeating Depression

Tranquility does not have to come from drugs. Stress and working in one position causes tenseness of the muscles. Scientists have found that a brisk fifteen-minute walk will do more for tense muscles than both a tranquilizer and a muscle relaxant. The relaxant effect of exercise can help a person sleep better. The sleep that exercise provides is a deep, healthy kind that refreshes both the body and mind.

If you are fighting a battle with depression, exercise can help you win. Depression affects everyone at some time or another. The feelings of helplessness that accompany depression frequently paralyze people with inactivity.

Exercise combats this helplessness by making you take action. Walking around the block, playing a competitive game of tennis, or working out in an aerobics class revitalizes your body and the way you think. Exercise makes you feel good because you are taking a definite action that is beneficial to your body.

Taking those first few steps toward exercise when you don't even feel like moving is never easy. But if you'll make yourself go for a walk, you'll begin to break the vicious hold of depression. Start walking a short distance then increase it each day. When you succeed in one area, you'll want to go on to another. You can lick depression without drugs.

More Energy for You

Exercise can increase your energy. I actually have *more* energy after I have exercised than before. This is caused by the endorphins provided by the brain when we exercise. Not much is known about these chemicals except that they seem to act as a pain killer or mood lifter. Endorphins seem to kill the pain of exercising and leave one with a happy, calm feeling for several hours after exercise.

Some people call this the "runner's high." But to me it means more energy to work and think. Lack of exercise will make you feel run down and give you symptoms very similar to an iron deficiency. In fact, researchers believe lack of exercise will not only drain your energy but help bring on disease. If you feel too tired to do anything after work and the doctor can find nothing wrong with you, try exercising and see if your energy does not shortly return.

Even more recent studies have shown that exercisers produce their own internal protein, known as *interlenkin 1*, that helps strengthen the body's ability to fight disease. This substance may explain why exercisers are generally more healthy than inactive people, experiencing fewer colds, sprains, strains, and accidents.

Some research shows that exercise raises the level of HDL, or good cholesterol. Researchers compared HDL levels in thirty-five postal carriers with those in inactive men. The level of HDL was higher in mailmen. The steady, regular, daily walking of the mailmen seemed to be responsible for the rise in HDL. Doctors believe you can reduce the risk of disease by being moderately active each day. You don't have to be a marathoner to be healthy. Walking regularly will reap tremendous benefits for your body and life.

The Wonder Drug

The benefits of exercise could fill a whole book. Following is a general summary of some of the main points:

1. Lowers serum cholesterol levels in the blood.
2. Lowers blood pressure.
3. Improves muscle tone in the legs thereby reducing the ill-effects of varicose veins.
4. Lowers blood sugar. (Research has shown that exercise improves the body's ability to metabolize sugar for about twelve hours. Therefore, diabetics should exercise at least three to four times a week. Exercise may even help prevent diabetes or certainly reduce its effect).
5. Strengthens bones and helps in preventing calcium deficiencies.
6. Wards off arthritis by keeping joints mobile.
7. Enables restful sleep.
8. Increases oxygen to the brain resulting in clearer thinking.

9. Improves sense of self-worth and general well-being.
10. Improves skin tone and slows the aging process of skin.
11. Increases body's ability to absorb nutrients.
12. Strengthens heart, lungs and other internal organs.
13. Decreases pain.
14. Lowers the body's set point (the weight your body seeks to maintain).
15. Decreases appetite.
16. Lengthens life span. (Exercisers live an average of three years longer than non-exercisers).
17. Encourages self-discipline.
18. Helps burn calories up to twenty-four hours after exercising.
19. Improves body's ability to fight disease by stimulating the immune system.
20. Burns fat while building muscle.
21. Increases stamina.

Nature's Diet Pill

Besides giving you a more youthful metabolism, vigorous exercise also serves as an appetite suppressant. Have you ever noticed that it is sometimes an hour or more after exercise before you are hungry? Have you also noticed that the more inactive you become, the more you want to eat?

Exercise cuts the appetite because it helps release fat into your blood stream, which stabilizes your blood sugar level. A drop in blood sugar triggers hunger, but exercise can keep hunger pangs away by maintaining a good level of blood sugar.

The numerous physical, emotional, and psychological benefits of exercise outweigh the initial aches and pains that accompany the start of most exercise programs. Remember to select an activity that you enjoy, start gradually, and pace yourself whenever you increase the intensity or duration of your program.

Anyone who will commit a portion of each day to exercise will never regret that decision. Be consistent and don't get discouraged if results are not immediate. A leaner, firmer, healthier you is just around the corner.

18

Getting the Most Out of Exercise

Many doctors have instructed their patients to start exercising but never told them how to start, what to do, and how long to do it. That's where health coaches like me can be of help.

Begin your exercise program by finding a health coach who can show you how to exercise. Start slowly for perhaps ten or fifteen minutes a day. Over the next six to eight weeks, gradually work up to thirty minutes of exercise at least three times each week.

Should you experience pain in the chest, dizziness, nausea or unusual loss of breath, consult your physician at once. Don't overdo. Breathe deeply as you go. Exercise until you are comfortably tired—not totally exhausted.

During my TV program, I don't count out the exercises so the viewer can go at her own pace. I use soft music as a background to sooth and ease any tensions the exerciser, especially the new exerciser, may be feeling. But even beginners need to exercise until it begins to "burn" a little. Exercise each part of your body that you can. Remember, if you don't use it, you lose it!

Exercise does not mean floating around in a pool or sweating in a hot tub. It is not walking ten blocks and then stopping for a hot fudge sundae at the corner ice cream store. Exercise is not just lifting weights.

Aerobic exercises, which include walking, cycling, aerobic dancing, jumping rope, and rowing, do the most to burn fat. To be beneficial, exercise must take place at least three times a week for at least thirty to forty-five minutes. Every day is best. My exercise program includes working on body alignment, arms, waist, abdomen, lower back, inner thighs, hips, and thighs.

The word *aerobic* means "with oxygen." Aerobic exercise is any exercise that requires the body to use large amounts of oxygen and requires the large muscles of the body to work in a continuous fashion for twenty minutes or more.

To be effective, exercise must go on long enough to put the pulse into its "target zone"—that area where your heart beats fast enough and long enough to afford you the maximum benefit. To find your target zone subtract your age from 220. Multiply the result by 70 percent and then by 85 percent. The resulting numbers show you the range in which your heart should beat during exercise.

Effective Exercise

If you want to add to the effectiveness of your exercising, never miss a chance to walk or climb stairs. You are doing yourself a favor when you take the stairs instead of the escalator. If you can walk instead of ride, great. Walking is a cardiovascular exercise and greatly benefits the heart.

How effective your exercise is depends to a great extent on your size to begin with. Heavier people burn more calories than thinner ones while doing the same exercises. Colder air enables you to burn more calories. Obviously, the harder you work, the more calories you will burn.

Some people like to add weights to their floor exercises or aerobic exercises. This is fine if you know what you're doing. One woman began to experience pain in her lower back, shoulders, and knees when she added weights to her aerobic workout. These side-effects may happen when a person tries to add too much weight too quickly. Start with one-pound weights and increase them gradually over a period of several months.

Many exercises are relatively safe for people with back problems. Discuss your alternatives with your doctor. Certainly walking and biking are safe for most people. Swimming and many floor exercises can be added to your routine without harm.

If you are experiencing pain at any point during exercise, then slow down or stop and rest. There may very well be some exercises you simply cannot do. You must heed your body when it warns you with pain. Serious injury can result if you do not.

Exercising when you are angry or greatly anxious can have negative effects on your blood pressure and circulation.

Everyone can learn to exercise. No one is hopeless. You may feel awkward at first, but the benefits are endless. You will find a regular exercise program improves your self-esteem and even changes your whole life. When you exercise your body, you uplift your spirit. We want hard bodies and soft hearts.

Which Exercise is Best?

I am often asked whether running or swimming is the best exercise. Research has shown that running usually burns more calories than swimming and will lead to quicker weight loss. But do the one that you enjoy. If you hate to run, chances are you will not run enough to lose weight. If you love to swim, swim. Doing an exercise that you like is necessary if you are going to stick to it long enough to accomplish anything.

Rowing is an excellent way to burn 1,000 calories an hour. This little-known exercise works many muscles including the upper body, arms, back, and legs. To maximize the calorie-burning aspect of a rowing machine, row slowly for thirty minutes or more at least three times a week. Rowing faster will increase your heart performance, but tiring sooner will result in less total calories being burned. Row slowly, and row as long as you can, as often as you can.

If you burn 2,000 calories a week, you will live longer. How much exercise does it take to burn 2,000 calories in one week? You can jog seventeen miles, play five hours of tennis, four hours of racquetball, ride a bike for three and one-half hours, or swim four hours.

Is Jogging for Everyone?

A woman who was fifty pounds overweight wrote to a doctor who specializes in sports medicine, asking him if she should jog to lose her excess poundage. She wanted to know if she might injure her feet or legs. The doctor replied that she was definitely not a candidate for jogging.

With each step, running can place as much as 400 to 1,000 pounds of stress on the feet of a person of average weight. For the overweight person the stress would be considerably more, resulting in inevitable injuries.

For the person who can jog, running can increase bone density without wearing out knees, hips, and ankles. Running can be very relaxing and an excellent way to deal with stress. Studies have shown that running can have a very positive psychological effect. Just don't become so absorbed in running that you neglect your family or other important areas of your life as some people have been known to do. Exercise moderation in all things.

If you jog, wear only absorbent fabrics such as cotton knits. Avoid vinyl, rubber, and plastics. They can throw the body's thermostat out of kilter and prevent natural body cooling. Wear fabrics that allow the skin to breath.

Jogging: Benefits and Risks

Here's what running can do for you:

1. Makes your circulatory system more efficient and thus gives you more energy.
2. Usually lowers the level of low-density lipoproteins (LDL) in the blood. (LDL, known as the "bad cholesterol," sticks to artery walls and can cause heart disease and death).
3. Strengthens heart ventricles so your heart does not have to beat as often to pump the blood.
4. Enhances shape and strength of legs.
5. Usually increases the level of "good cholesterol," or high-density lipoproteins (HDL) in the blood.
6. Aids in weight loss.

Running burns about 100 calories per mile, no matter how fast or slow you go. If you walk a mile or run it, you will burn about the same number of calories. Running, as with all aerobic exercising, will aid in burning calories and will increase your metabolism even after you've finished.

Runners always burn a mixture of carbohydrates and fats. Running within two hours after a meal will tend to burn more fat. If you run earlier, you will be more likely to burn carbohydrates.

You can run too much and risk serious injury. Here are some signs of overdoing it:

1. Muscle tenderness to the touch.
2. Unusual fatigue during a run.
3. Depression, irritability, and anxiety.
4. Insomnia or frequent waking.
5. Elevated resting heart rate.

These symptoms will occur before the evidence of injury manifests itself. They are a warning to you to rest more and reduce your mileage. If pain occurs, don't run. See your doctor. Never run during periods of high humidity.

Attitude and Exercise

One viewer wrote, "My goal is to fit into jeans with pockets. I have a way to go but am down one size in three weeks."

In weight loss and in exercise, attitude counts as much as anything. "Wanting" to exercise because you know what it can do for you will help you do a better job and do it more consistently. Setting goals also helps you stick with an exercise program.

On my exercise program I try to make each viewer feel like an important person. In order to make exercise an important part of your day, you must like yourself and be willing to work hard. I never knew anyone who "fell" into fitness. You can't play at exercise. There are no short cuts.

I like to talk to myself when I am exercising alone. The encouragement works wonders. I tell myself, "You're doing great. Come on, just a little bit longer. You can do it. You're going to look great in that new dress!"

Along with positive self-talk, a technique called dissociation has also been helpful to me. *Dissociation* is focusing your mind on things other than what your body is experiencing during exercise. Thinking about a field of flowers or a flowing stream or anything that is pleasant will carry you through the exercises. This technique can help you in other areas of your life that may be stressful or unpleasant. The Scriptures encourage us to do something similar:

> Finally, brothers, whatever is true, whatever is noble, whatever is right, whatever is pure, whatever is lovely, whatever is admirable—if anything is excellent or praiseworthy—think about such things—Philippians 4:8, NIV.

Your endurance and performance in life and in exercise often hinges on your thought patterns. A positive outlook and belief in God and what God can do through you is a wonderful way to face any challenge. The Lord has promised us a glorified body in heaven, but He has told us to take care of this body while we are on earth. When you take care of your body, you are doing a godly thing.

Warming Up

Exercise progresses more smoothly when you warm up or build up to a full exercise level, especially if you are doing something as demanding as aerobics or jogging. Sudden change in heart rate, like that brought on by just jumping into an aerobic dance session, can trigger a heart attack. A gradual acceleration of the heart rate is best. Warm-ups also gradually increase body temperature, enhancing the flexibility of tendons and the muscles' ability to contract and relax.

Warm-ups bring your muscles to the point where they can best exercise. When you are at rest, 85 percent of your blood supply is in the abdomen and chest. As activity begins, blood supply shifts to the muscles. After six to ten minutes of activity, you are ready to work out.

The safest way to reach the work-out stage is to do a low-intensity activity. For example, joggers can start with a slow, easy shuffle. Aerobics people can begin with a brisk walk. Never stretch without warming up first. You can tear muscle if you do.

Cooling Down

Ending your time of exercise correctly is just as important as beginning it correctly. To suddenly stop exercising without tapering off is to risk a post-workout heart attack.

The American Medical Association reports that men who exercise hard and then suddenly stop may experience an increase in a hormone that can trigger irregular heartbeats. Research shows that the first two or three minutes after any vigorous exercise are critical. Walk around during the cooldown period to give the heart time to adjust.

Dr. Kenneth Cooper, director of the Dallas-based Aerobics Center, surmised that the heart attack that killed fitness expert Jim Fixx could have been caused by his stopping at an intersection. Continuing to jog in place as he waited for the light to change could have prevented his fatal heart attack.

Vigorous exercise creates a demand for large volumes of blood to be delivered to working muscles. If activity is suddenly halted, the heart will not slow down immediately. The heart continues to pump blood to the muscles that were being used up until a moment ago. As large amounts of blood continue to flood the muscles, the brain may not get enough blood. This can bring on fainting. If the heart is not getting enough blood, the exerciser could have a heart attack.

At the end of a horserace, thoroughbreds make a full circle of the track before stopping. People must do the same thing—taper off before stopping. How long should you cool down? Until your breathing returns to normal and your pulse is no longer pounding.

What About Saunas and Other "Therapies"?

Saunas, whirlpools, and steam rooms provide good ways to relax after a workout. Many people enjoy them more for socializing than for their health benefits. There are advantages and disadvantages to their use, however.

Dry sauna heat will allow you to sweat off 17 fluid ounces of water and toxic minerals in a single session while burning as much as 300 calories. Steam room heat will relax tight muscles and soothe sore joints. The fluid lost in both these methods is only temporary and is soon replaced.

Whirlpools are relaxing but they contain health risks as do saunas and steam rooms. Hot tubs that are not properly maintained can spread bacteria, herpes, and even a mild form of Legionnaires' disease.

For people with a history of heart attacks, the saunas and steam rooms are extremely dangerous because the stress of the sudden temperature change can bring on an attack. Every time you change temperature in any direction, your heart rate increases. In high temperatures, the blood pressure will drop. For people who suffer from arteriosclerosis, such a sudden drop could bring on a stroke.

Whether or not you go for the saunas, whirlpools, or steam rooms after a workout should depend on your general health and on whether the facilities are sanitary and properly maintained. If you have already perspired a lot in your workout, it may be foolish to risk more fluid loss. The heat could dry out your skin too much.

If you choose to use these therapies, limit your time to six minutes if you are new at it or fifteen minutes if you are accustomed to it. After you finish, drink plenty of water or fruit juice to replace lost fluid. Shower and shampoo thoroughly to remove salts and chemicals from your pores and moisturize your skin. Consult with your physician before you use these therapies, especially if you are pregnant, on medication, or experiencing any health problems.

Sweating it Out

Sweating is a natural process and an essential part of exercise. As we exercise our bodies heat up. We sweat to cool off. Perspiration is the body's cooling system.

The taller or heavier you are the more you will sweat. This is because tall and heavy people have less skin surface per unit of weight.

Don't expect to stop perspiring as soon as you stop exercising. Our bodies gradually cool down and will continue to perspire for as long as the temperature remains above normal.

There is no truth to the myth that one must shower immediately after exercise or the perspiration will clog the pores and cause skin problems like acne. In fact, showering before you have cooled down is useless because your body will continue to perspire even after showering. Perspiration is a good way to clear the pores.

What *will* irritate the skin is too much showering. Over-showering causes rough, dry skin. Showers wash away surface oils that keep the skin moist and supple. Soap dries skin so badly that it should be a habit with you to moisturize after every shower.

The major problem with sweating is not sweating enough. In the course of one hour of exercise, your body can become overheated if you do not perspire. Be sure to drink water as you exercise to aid the body in its cooling efforts.

What Your Body Needs

Increasing your physical activity will not necessarily mean you will need to change your diet or increase your nutrient intake. If you eat a balanced diet you will not necessarily need to take vitamins either. The only supplement you may need would be iron. This is particularly true for menstruating women.

If you are already thin but you want to continue a regular exercise program, you may have to increase your caloric intake or risk becoming too thin. Few people have this problem, but some do. Any increase in calories should be in the form of complex carbohydrates.

Recent research has shown that exercise does raise your body's need for riboflavin or vitamin B-2. A deficiency in riboflavin will cause lips to split at the corners of the mouth; eyes will burn, itch, and tire easily; headaches and swallowing difficulties will develop.

Since riboflavin plays a big role in maintaining energy levels and in keeping your eyes and skin healthy, it must be carefully monitored. Riboflavin also plays an important role in metabolism of carbohydrates, fats, and protein.

Women who exercise should be sure to add riboflavin-rich foods to their diets. Supplements should be taken only at your doctor's recommendation. Milk is the best source of riboflavin. Since B-2 is destroyed by light, buy milk in the light-proof containers. Other riboflavin-rich foods include yogurt, oysters, black beans, asparagus, broccoli, collards, mushrooms, brewer's yeast, and wild rice.

Water Workouts

Water is an ideal medium for relieving pain and stiffness for anyone having difficulty moving muscles and joints, whether from an accident, surgery, stroke or disease. Because your body is almost weightless in water, the pull of gravity on sore or deformed joints is minimal and your range of motion is greater than on dry land.

At the same time the active resistance of the water strengthens and tones your muscles. With arthritic pain, muscles will waste away if not used. A planned program of gentle, controlled stretching and limbering movements in water can stop or at least slow down the pain and crippling in severe cases. You don't need to know how to swim to benefit from water exercises.

Exercise Footnotes

Have you ever experienced a "stitch" in your side when exercising? Most of us have. What causes that sudden pain? The respiratory muscles may not be getting enough oxygen. The problem seems to be particularly worse in people who have stopped exercising for a while and then go back in full force. Improper, rapid, shallow breathing appears to be the cause.

The best way to get rid of a stitch is to stop exercising so that the blood supply can catch up with the blood demand. Blow air out as hard as you can to empty the air from your lungs, then inhale fully. Stretching the arm over your head on the side that hurts should also relieve some of the pain.

Soreness is especially a problem when you first begin exercising. Regular exercisers do not get sore. Why?

A protein that is crucial to the healing process continually circulates in the bloodstream of well-trained exercisers. In one university study a group of athletes and a group of inactive people were tested on a bicycle that was especially rigged to work muscles that are used when running downhill.

After exercise, the athletes were less sore because of the high levels of this protein in their muscles. The protein floods into the bloodstream of the inactive group only after exercise has occurred. The muscles of a regular exerciser are geared up for healing and are constantly repairing themselves.

A warm bath after a workout will help ease soreness. If you do become sore, don't work quite as hard until the soreness begins to leave. But do continue to work out. When soreness leaves, you know you are building lean muscle mass.

Use It or Lose It

Suppose I've convinced you to begin exercising regularly and you diligently follow a program for six months or even a year. Then your husband gets a promotion and you have to pack up and move to another state. Or your mother-in-law comes to visit for a month or two. Something happens, and you get out of the habit of exercise.

One day you look in the mirror and those beautiful, firm thighs that you had a few weeks ago are beginning to look like the surface of the moon. What happened? If you stop working out, muscles will begin to disappear and they will be replaced by fat or cellulite.

Amino acids move in and out of the muscles all the time and they make the muscles strong. Exercise serves as a stimulus to keep these acids going back into the muscles. If we don't exercise regularly, the acids are sent to the liver and later excreted. The result—loss of muscle tissue.

Body Alignment

To get the maximum benefit from exercise, a person should have proper body alignment—or the proper positioning of the head and body in an upward direction and the inhibiting of unnecessary muscle movement.

Body alignment is what any good ballet or modern dance instructor would teach you. Train yourself to pay attention to posture in your day-by-day life.

Benefits of having proper body alignment include:

1. Improvement of appearance.
2. Greater benefit from exercise;
3. Better sleep.
4. More energy.
5. Relief of pain and pressure in the lower back.
6. Better sense of balance.

The most obvious benefit is the way it improves your appearance. After a few lessons in posture, it is quite common for someone to look five to ten pounds thinner without having lost a pound.

Many women have a problem with their lower back being swayed too much. Under stress the shoulder, waist, and lower back muscles will ache. When a person is not aligned in the most efficient way, she will tend to overstress her joints.

Making change in posture is not easy. Posture tends to become fixed with age. For example, slouching in your office chair can affect how you hold yourself all the time.

Slouching tightens the upper body muscles, making your chest cave in. Supporting muscles in your upper back become weak and stretched out and thus fail to keep the shoulders back. If you allow this to continue, slumping becomes your only option.

Along with body alignment, a person must learn to breath more deeply. Not only do you bring more air into your body by breathing deeply, but deep breathing also helps release over-all tension.

I read of one woman who, as a child and in her teens, was so flexible she could do cartwheels, splits, and roll herself into a ball. But by her early thirties something had happened. Some of this "folding" became permanent. Her shoulders became rounded and her chest caved in somewhat. She was tall and her lower back swayed in too much and her hip muscles were too tight. Her shoulder, waist, and lower back muscles began to ache. Medical experts told her she was heading for chronic back trouble.

She began an exercise program that taught body alignment. The stress on her joints was eased and in a few weeks people were asking her if she had lost weight. She had not lost a pound, but she looked thinner because of her improved posture.

Investing in Your Life Span

Your health requires a total commitment from you. No price tag can be placed on it. Good health takes time, patience, nurturing, and commitment.

Look at your diet and exercise commitment as an investment in your life span. No, it isn't going to be easy. But the increased energy, productivity, self-worth, well-being, improved appearance, and reduction in trips to the doctor make it worthwhile.

Part Four
You and Your Health

19

Are You a Food Addict?

Mary was a chronic dieter. Even when dieting, thoughts of food consumed her waking hours. She compared her problem to that of an alcoholic, drug addict, or gambler, and she was right. Mary was a food addict.

Food addiction and overeating are not the same thing. Overeating does not necessarily mean you are addicted to food. We all overeat at times. Overeating is caused by an abundance of food, how good it is, and how much variety there is. If you've ever gone to a buffet, you probably ate much more than you normally would at an ordinary meal.

Food addiction is a much more serious matter. The food addict can think of nothing else but food. She spends a lot of time just deciding what to eat next. Like smoking and drinking, food addiction is both psychological and physical in nature.

Feeling compelled to eat, a food addict often cannot stop even when she wants to. Eating is a comfort to her—it seems to fill all the hurting and lonely places in her life. What makes food addiction worse than other addictions, however, is that no one can completely stop eating. A food addict must re-train her thinking and learn to eat in moderation and for the right reasons.

Am I a Compulsive Overeater?

Ask yourself these questions if you think you may have a problem with food abuse: "When I eat, do I eat because I am hungry? Do I taste the food? Do I remember what I ate and how much?"

Less than 5 percent of the population of the United States are truly compulsive overeaters. Eating instead of writing a term paper or cleaning the garage, for example, does not necessarily mean you are a compulsive overeater. You may simply dread a certain job.

A true compulsive overeater is obsessed with eating and cannot control the urge. It's not a matter of eating until satisfied and then stopping. It is a matter of eating and eating and not being able to stop.

The compulsive overeater is not even bulimic. The bulimic decides to binge and knows exactly what she is doing. She goes to the market and buys food and plans to binge on it. The compulsive overeater hardly realizes food has been eaten or even what was eaten.

Conquering the Compulsion

An overeater should have nothing to do with fad or crash diets. Instead, the food addict should search for a good health coach who can instruct her in good eating habits and healthy exercise. That will do more than all the diets in the world. A Christian counselor, pastor or friend who will pray, listen, and point the sufferer to God's love and care is invaluable.

Start by giving up self-pity. Let go of the past and its failures. Learn to take problems to the Lord and trust in His love and care. He loves us and thinks we are wonderful. As we get to know Him more, His love will begin to heal all the broken places in our lives and fill any emptiness we may feel.

Combining a close relationship with the Lord with a balanced diet and good exercise is the victory formula for any person suffering with substance abuse. God cares about the food abuser and He wants to see them set free from their bondage.

Weather and Overeating

Overeating is caused by a variety of factors, and some are more surprising than others. A study on weather and how it affects weight has revealed some interesting data.

1. Even when sticking to a diet and exercise regimen, you can expect to see a weight increase when a cold front passes through. The body loses less water through evaporation.
2. Some appetites, especially those of women, tend to be influenced by the weather. For example, some people drastically cut food intake during hot weather and also tend to eat more fresh fruits and vegetables during this time.
3. Bad winter-time weather leads to weight gain. If a winter storm approaches, people rush out to stock up on essentials and goodies. Then when they are housebound and bored, they eat more.
4. Exercise in cold air leads to greater weight loss. Calories are burned as the body tries to keep warm.
5. Mood is affected by weather. If gloomy weather depresses you and if you eat when you are depressed, you will eat more during gloomy weather. Knowing this can help us learn to control our eating better during these times.

Other Causes of Overeating

Both emotional and biochemical factors affect appetite. One survey revealed that people eat to relieve tension. Eaters are not seeking a full stomach or even the taste of food, but are seeking the relief that comes from chewing. Research is being done to make a low-calorie chew bar for stressed overeaters to gnaw.

Studies have shown that many overweight people need more variety, aroma, texture, and taste to their food than the average person. If deprived of these factors, they will overeat continually in search of fulfillment. Such people have responded well to diets with lots of "crunch" added to them—like carrots and celery.

Some people overeat simply because they are over-responding to food cues. You've probably heard these people lament, "I can just look at food, and I will gain weight."

As these people watched food cooking, their blood showed remarkably higher levels of insulin than the average person. Insulin has a definite impact on appetite. For those who over-respond to food cues, the answer is to take a brisk walk or drink a glass of water.

Do You Crave Carbohydrates?

Studies have shown that some people overeat because they have an inborn craving for carbohydrates. These people always have a taste for cake, candy, and other simple carbohydrates. Researchers say that eating carbohydrates raises the level of serotonin, a neurotransmitter in the brain that produces a sense of being satisfied or full.

The craving for carbohydrates subsides if suitable forms are included in each meal. When these people go on a low-carbohydrate diet, however, they begin to feel irritable. Their intense craving for carbohydrates often results in binging on sweets until they are sick.

The answer? A high-complex carbohydrate diet that is low in fat will maintain nutritional balance. An occasional sweet to satisfy the craving is better than total abstinence followed by binging.

Two things can trigger a sweets binge—total abstinence for too long a time or just one bite of something sweet.

You have to know yourself. If you have a problem with craving sweets, find out what works for you. Some people have to stay away from sweets completely, or they will binge. Others are better able to avoid binging if they allow themselves a sweet from time to time.

Who is a Chocoholic?

Many people say they are chocoholics when they aren't. Enjoying chocolate is different from using chocolate to deal with stress. The chocoholic is like a food addict—he deals with stress by eating, except he prefers chocolate.

Those who deal with stress by eating chocolate are really suffering. Eating chocolate serves the same purpose as taking a drink or a tranquilizer. Very few people, however, are really hooked on chocolate.

Sometimes people tell me they are chocoholics. They often say, "I see my family eating sweets and I have to have some. How in the world will I ever be able to discipline myself?"

All you ever have to do is exercise. Commit that time to your health. As you exercise and develop discipline in that area of your life, it will carry over into your eating. You will find yourself looking at food and calculating its nutritional value. Desiring energy for your body, you'll ask, "Why should I do all this work and turn around and ruin it all with a poor diet?"

Discipline carries right down the line. When you discipline yourself in one area, you are better able to control other areas of your life. If you've spent an hour exercising, you'll think twice before indulging yourself and adding 900 unwanted calories to your hips.

Foods and Moods

Do you find yourself craving chocolate or diving into the cookie jar when you're feeling depressed, irritable, anxious, afraid, bored, or maybe just lonely? Many women crave carbohydrates the week prior to menstruation. Doctors have found a correlation between mild depression and binges on simple carbohydrates such as cakes and cookies.

Does the mood cause the craving, or is the craving a result of the mood? Do you choose what to eat, or does your mood choose for you? While you have no control over your biological drive to eat, you do have control over how you handle that drive.

Research has shown that emotional conditions such as fear, tension, boredom, and loneliness can very strongly influence what we want to eat. People have different food cravings because they need different foods to alter their feelings. A lot of work has been done to show the relationship between carbohydrates and depression.

As a result of complex chemical reactions inside the body, some foods are mood boosters while others are mood bombs. Why is this?

When you eat large amounts of straight carbohydrates, you increase the brain's production of a chemical that affects appetite, pain, and alertness. The connection between depression and a deficiency in this chemical is very strong. Some scientists believe a deficiency in this chemical can cause depression.

Dealing with Depression

One study showed that as certain women became depressed they ate more carbohydrates; when the depression lifted, they ate fewer carbohydrates. Researchers feel these women may have subconsciously been using carbohydrates as a form of self-medication to relieve their depression. They craved carbohydrates because they had learned from experience that eating them eased depression.

Even though we may know why we crave carbohydrates, let's not binge on them to cure the blues! Even though snacking on carbohydrates may temporarily ease depression, binging on them will only lead to obesity. The fat you eat is the fat you wear. The price you pay for a temporary lift to your spirits will also show up on your bathroom scales.

Instead of binging on simple, sugary carbohydrates, try a more natural approach to health and happiness. Exercise will release endorphins, the body's natural mood elevator, and burn calories as well. Complex carbohydrates such as fresh fruits and vegetables, low-fat cheeses, and yogurts will boost your spirits and keep you from gaining weight.

Emotional Hunger

For the true food addict, food is a way of dealing with mental pain and discomfort. Food actually provides relief from distress rather than nourishment or pleasure. A trip to the refrigerator becomes an escape from problems. Like other addictions, food cannot eradicate the real problems. Food addiction hurts relationships with others, lowers self-esteem, and creates health problems.

Inevitably the food addict hits "rock bottom" when he decides his overeating must stop—that he cannot continue shoveling in food and abusing his body. This moment may come while hiding in the pantry or in the bathroom as he's cramming down a whole cake or a pizza. The mind is screaming with self-hatred and crying for help.

One characteristic of virtually all food addicts is that they or their parents (or both) have unrealistic goals and expectations of what is considered "good" and "commendable" behavior. These people tend to be on a never-fulfilled search for approval and acceptance. They are always striving for some elusive idea of perfection that has been imposed on them by their parents or by some factor within themselves.

Although these people tend to be very talented and intelligent, they never feel successful even when they should.

Nothing is ever enough to convince them of their worth. Their sparkling, clean house always looks dirty and inferior to them. Despite being straight A students, they still feel like failures. These tortured individuals constantly stretch themselves to their limits of mental and physical endurance. Ultimately they are always frustrated and unhappy. They take comfort in food.

Food cannot make anything better. Over-indulging in food will only mask the processes of your inner life. After eating compulsively you are still faced with whatever emotional turmoil triggered your eating in the first place. Emotions are not monsters or objects. They are quite simply a part of you—even the dreadfully painful ones. And you have to face them.

People often eat to cover hurts, not realizing they would experience greater relief in dealing with their personal pain than expending so much energy trying to suppress them. Allowing negative feelings to surface enables you to deal with them. Feelings are not meant to be alleviated but rather experienced. Once you recognize and face your feelings, they will become less frightening.

Stress and Food Addiction

If you have developed an addiction to food, you are not alone. You are vulnerable to such problems because of the stressful life you live. Being a wife, mother, friend; balancing a career with homemaking; trying to remain slim and healthy—all these pressures cause us to become overloaded.

If you have ways to combat stress, such as exercising daily, eating well-balanced meals, and making sure you get a good night's sleep, then all will be well. But if you have no mechanisms to combat stress, watch out! You may be tempted to fall back on what is handy and very often that is food.

Food has been your comfort in the past. You can remember Mom giving you cookies and milk when you fell down and bumped your knee. Food was used to combat stress and take your mind off your troubles.

Many people have been entangled in food addictions by substituting food for proper coping mechanisms. Addiction means relying on food to solve your problems. If you feel lonely, ashamed, angry, confused or empty, you get something to eat. Afterwards, for a brief time, you may feel better—perhaps quieter, calmer, more satisfied. But when troubled thoughts return, you seek food for comfort and relief. Before you know it, a vicious cycle has begun.

Hormones and Eating Disorders

The brain reacts two ways to long-term stress and depression. First, it causes increased levels of the hormone CRF, which affects appetite. People who suffer from depression and anorexia have increased levels of this hormone. Second, long-term stress over-stimulates the nervous system and exhausts its supply of neurotransmitters which, in turn, increases depression. (Neurotransmitters are chemicals that carry messages between nerve cells.)

The release of the CRF hormone affects the monthly cycle in women and can cause them to cease menstruating. CRF is also the reason anorexics can exercise for hours and hours, abusing their bodies without even feeling it.

On the other hand, stress can cause just the opposite reactions in people and lead to bulimia and obesity. The brain releases beta-endorphins that cause a craving for carbohydrates and sweets; the subsequent binge creates a false euphoria within the bulimic or obese person.

This is why bulimics and obese persons eat such great amounts of sweets and other carbohydrates—they truly *do* experience a short-lived sense of well-being. But the euphoria quickly leaves, and the sufferer lives in a hellish cycle of stress and overeating.

What the Brain Craves

The type of food we eat affects certain neurotransmitters in the brain that regulate appetite. One neurotransmitter in particular, serotonin, controls how much you eat as well as your body's desire for protein and carbohydrates. Low levels of serotonin can cause people to eat too much and to eat the wrong foods as well.

When food is digested, it is broken down into nutrients, including amino acids. Tryptophan is an amino acid that is the main building material for serotonin. Foods rich in tryptophan will increase serotonin in the brain and enable your brain to inform you that you are full. Fluctuation in the serotonin will also tell your body which foods to eat.

If you listen to your body, you will naturally eat a balanced diet. When you eat complex carbohydrates or simple carbohydrates (sweets), your serotonin level increases. You will feel full and at your next meal will crave protein, which will lower the serotonin levels. At your next meal you will want carbohydrates again. To keep serotonin levels on track, follow a balanced diet.

Food Allergies

In some cases food abuse is a result of food allergies. Being allergic to certain foods can cause cravings for those foods and can lead to weight gain and binging.

In most cases, allergic reactions are visible with wheezing, running nose, and teary eyes. With food allergies, reactions vary from diarrhea, bloating of the abdomen, vomiting, and constipation. Certain foods can cause migraine headaches. As many as one in five Americans may suffer from migraine headaches. Headaches can be brought on by factors other than food allergies, but food allergies account for many.

If you experience migraines and do not know why, try keeping a diary of the foods you ate prior to the attack.

By process of elimination, you may be able to discover if your headache is caused by something you are eating.

The foods most commonly associated with migraines are milk, coffee, tea, colas, citrus fruits, grapes, nuts, legumes, yeast, pineapple, coconut, wheat, pork, chocolate, beef, and cane sugar. Chemical additives in such foods as cured meats, cheeses, and alcoholic beverages can also cause a migraine attack.

If you suspect that your overeating may be caused by food allergies, make an appointment with an allergist who will be able to tell you exactly what you are allergic to. The offending food is usually a food you like and eat often. The three most common culprits in causing allergies are wheat, corn, and milk.

I know one alert mother who, through her own process of elimination, discovered that whole wheat bread led to an endless round of ear infections in her child. When the child stopped eating the whole wheat bread, the ear problem cleared up.

Most of the time maintaining balance and moderation in diet along with regular exercise will greatly alleviate allergy problems.

As for whether or not food allergies lead to overeating and food abuse, there is little scientific evidence to support this theory. Again, experts feel that fad dieting and stress lead to food abuse and binge eating.

Obesity—The Tragic Result

You are obese if you weigh 20 percent more than is desirable for your height. Obesity is a disease that can increase risk of death. But even carrying five to ten extra pounds can put a person at a higher risk of high blood pressure or diabetes.

Because of their extra fat, obese people triple their risk of developing hypertension, double the risk of high cholesterol, and triple the risk of diabetes. The increased risks come from the way fat alters the body's metabolism and biochemical functioning, wearing down the body's natural defenses to the point where they break and disease results.

New studies have shown that overeating simple carbohydrates such as candy, potato chips, and soda pop forces the heart to pump harder. The extra load on the heart makes it more susceptible to failure or irregularities that may be linked to coronary heart disease.

Extra fat tissue also causes the body to resist its own insulin, leads to a wearing out of the pancreas, and increases the onset of diabetes. For every extra twenty pounds of body fat, an extra 200 milligrams of cholesterol are produced. This is concentrated in gallbladder bile and can eventually lead to gallstones. Obesity has been linked to arthritis in the knees and ankles, and to cancer of the uterus, breast, and prostate.

Whether you are bound by overeating or food addiction, the result will eventually be obesity if these disorders are not conquered. The dangerous diseases that are linked to being overweight should be motivation to trust the Lord for deliverance and victory over these abnormal cravings for food.

─────20─────
Bulimia and Anorexia

A few years ago I innocently got caught up in the "thinness" game. I was busy conducting exercise classes in several churches and going to the studio once a week to produce television programs. Students in my classes could not understand why I wasn't thinner—with all the exercise I was doing, I should be skin and bones.

Subconsciously, I wanted to please everyone. I started taking two sprigs of broccoli and half an apple with me for my lunch. I hardly ate anything at all and became compulsive about exercise.

Even if I taught two one-hour exercise classes and produced five shows in a day, I wasn't satisfied. At eight o'clock in the evening I would find myself back at the track to do my five-mile run or else at home feeling very blue because I had not followed my schedule that day.

One day I went to my exercise class at church feeling very good about myself because I weighed 93 pounds. I announced to the group of women, "Well, I hope I am thin enough for you. I weighed myself this morning, and my new low is 93 pounds." One of the ladies then said to me, "Beverly, you still aren't skinny."

Suddenly I knew I was on a path to self-destruction. I had started to become a "people pleaser" not a God pleaser. The results could have been tragic. I started thinking, "People will come to my funeral and say, 'Look at her. Why, she practically wasted away to nothing doing all that exercising. But you know something, she's still not skinny.' "

Precious person, don't let fashion or anything else do this to you. God showed me how wrong I was. Viewers who were bound by anorexia and bulimia had been sending me letters. Except for the grace of God, that could be me. I was on the verge of self-destruction. I thought, "How can I be a guide to others when I am so borderline sick myself?"

I made a commitment to God that a new balance would be sought in my life—God first, family second, and ministry third. I saw for the first time that obsession with eating and exercising are addictive and must be kept in proper balance.

Thin is In

Our society seems to equate thinness with success. Doctors caution against comparing your body to that of professional models, actors, and exercise experts. Culture's distorted idea of what a woman's shape should be has resulted in an increase in eating problems. Many women feel great pressure to starve themselves down to a size they were probably never meant to be.

Many scientists and doctors think our high-pressured society promotes the use of food crutches that lead to eating disorders such as anorexia, bulimia, and obesity. Most of the time these disorders first appear in early childhood when a child copes with family stresses like divorce or feelings of inferiority by using food for comfort. Many times a child controls and manipulates through food—not eating to get her way or overeating as an act of rebellion.

Starving for Attention

At the other end of extremes, many people deal with stress by not eating. A woman may begin the road to anorexia by wanting to lose only five pounds. After she loses that, she begins to take pride in the weight loss. Friends compliment her appearance. She loses another five pounds and receives more praise from her peers. She feels strong and capable—like she can do something others cannot do.

As she continues losing weight and receiving compliments, she overlooks the fact that she is dizzy, aches all over, and has a hard time getting her work done. Nothing is more important to her than losing weight.

Friends and family gradually begin to worry and ask her to stop losing weight. Instead of compliments, the anorexic's family tells her how bad she looks. She may try to stop, but many times it is already too late. What started as a *compulsion* has ended as an *addiction*. Something inside her has changed, and she can no longer see herself as she really is. She believes she is a fat, ugly girl who needs to lose more weight.

So what does she do? Her starvation diet causes her to flirt with death. Without proper nutrition, her kidneys, heart, or other vital organs will fail.

Anorexia Nervosa

Anorexia nervosa, which means "nervous loss of appetite," is misleading. Actually, the person afflicted with this disease thinks about food constantly but fights the urge to eat. An anorexic may take in as few as 300 to 600 calories per day. Anorexia is an emotional disease that results in malnutrition. A chemical deficiency in the brain triggers this biochemical disorder.

How can you recognize the anorexic? A weight loss of 15 to 25 percent of the pre-diet weight; compulsive and excessive exercise; unusual eating habits (denying hunger or eating only certain foods); heightened interest in recipes and cooking; preoccupation with dieting and calorie counting.

Anorexics are experts on calorie content. They are obsessed with their weight. As long as they're losing, they feel secure. But they will nearly always complain of feeling fat.

As the anorexic continues to starve herself, she will experience insomnia, constipation, dry skin, hair loss, weak and brittle nails, and a feeling of being cold all the time.

What's the difference between a starving person and an anorexic? A starving person will conserve energy by not moving about any more than necessary. The anorexic will usually be as compulsive about exercising as she is about not eating.

Anorexics fall into two categories—restricters and bulimics. *Restricters* do not binge or purge but severely limit their food intake. *Bulimics* starve themselves and binge eat. They consume large amounts of food and then purge the body by inducing vomiting or taking large doses of laxatives.

Bulimia may be more harmful than chronic starvation because it puts the body on a metabolic yo-yo. An anorexic victim denies that her behavior is wrong or harmful. A bulimic knows she is wrong but does not want to admit it.

What Causes Anorexia?

Why do bright, well-liked children go on diets and get so carried away they starve themselves to death? An alarming number of young women are reacting to the pressures of growing up by starving themselves. Parents play a key role in preventing and overcoming this disease.

Professionals tell us that anorexics may come from families that are insensitive to their emotional needs. When a girl feels ignored by parents who are too busy to listen, she looks for ways to gain attention. Perhaps she had previously been praised for her appearance or accomplishments.

The typical anorexic comes from an achievement-oriented family in which the child has few options or opportunities to control her own life. She learns that she can exert total control over food intake and weight.

When we tell a child we are counting on her to be the prettiest or the best, we are applying pressure and delivering a dreadful message that the child is not worthwhile unless she is the best. When a child cannot satisfy her parents' expectations, problems arise.

Another catalyst for anorexia is a family that is excessively conscious of body size. A child should never be criticized for her size or shape.

Helping The Anorexic

The incidence of anorexia nervosa is high, although many borderline cases go undiagnosed. Many anorexics are not in nutritional trouble. The first step in treating a dangerously anorexic young woman is *nutritional support.* She may require hospitalization and intravenous feeding.

The nutritional system has to be restored before psychological counseling can begin. While two to three months may be required to treat the nutritional problems, counseling may take much longer. Nutritional support may have to be repeated should the patient suffer a relapse into anorexic behavior.

The anorexic must learn proper eating habits. A balanced diet will help them avoid obesity, which would almost certainly trigger another bout with anorexia.

These diseases begin when a person is nagged about their weight. Hormonal changes during puberty can trigger problems. The emotional aspects of the disease make it hard to treat. Parents who see signs of it in a child should confront her in a loving, nonthreatening way and seek professional help immediately. A family physician can recommend specialists.

Bulimia—Out of Control

The following letter, sent to a doctor, is not uncommon. "Please help me. I am twenty years old, five feet, seven inches tall, and weigh about 145 pounds. I have been trying to lose weight all my life, and I am sick and tired of trying. The longest I have stayed on a diet is about four days. Then I get upset and start eating like there's no tomorrow. Afterward I throw up only to eat more food. I know it's disgusting but I can't stop. I'm depressed, and I cry myself to sleep. I can't tell my parents because they would get angry and tell me to stop. My boyfriend feels the same way. Please help me."

The doctors tell us this situation is not all that unusual. Most people who try to lose weight and can't, find themselves feeling angry, frustrated, and defeated. However, this young lady is out of control—she has bulimia.

Why is bulimia so common now? Our society is fixated on food, bodies, and the relentless pursuit of thinness! *The desire for absolute control or thinness gives bulimia its magic appeal!*

Profile of a Bulimic

The average bulimic is female, single, Caucasian, in her early twenties, educated, and of average weight. A bulimic consumes large amounts of simple carbohydrates in a relatively short time period (2,000 to 20,000 calories in two hours). Binges usually occur in the evening and almost always under private and secretive conditions.

The bulimic is aware of her disturbed eating pattern but is unable to stop binging. Because of her fear of gaining weight, she tries to be in rigid control. The real problem is that in allowing her life to be obsessed with the pursuit of thinness, she is really out of control.

Bulimics crave simple carbohydrates (cookies, cakes, and ice cream) because such foods help reduce psychic pain and discomfort from stress. When simple carbohydrates are eaten, the pancreas secretes insulin. In addition to aiding the digestion of sugar, insulin helps transport an amino acid (tryptophan) into the brain. Once in the brain, this substance is rapidly transformed into a powerful neurotransmitter (serotonin).

Increased levels of this hormone-like agent cause a feeling of calmness similar to that created by taking a mild tranquilizer. Resistance to pain and discomfort is also increased. This is the "binge calm" that follows the consumption of rich, sugar-laden foods. The binger feels a sense of relief and a temporary escape from problems and worries.

Binge, Purge, Relief

Binging on food to gain comfort or to avoid conflict is dangerous because the act becomes physically addictive. Once binging begins, it becomes more frequent until a true eating disorder such as compulsive eating, overeating, or bulimia occurs. The woman doing this feels she has *lost control*. She knows she is doing something *disgusting*.

After binging, the bulimic feels calmer, but she soon begins to feel guilty. Thinking about all those calories she has just consumed, she realizes how horribly fat she will become. When terror turns into panic, she tries to remove the offending food.

Self-induced vomiting, laxatives, and long, hard workouts are used to rid the body of unwanted calories. This is called purging. Just like binging, purging is dangerous and addictive. Many food addicts admit to purging to get rid of the food as well as the bad inner feelings (low self-esteem) that accompany overeating.

The purge actually sets the binger up for the next binge. Since purging actually rids the body of nutrients as well as food, the body soon sends out new hunger signals and the binger must eat again. Binging and purging is called *bulimia*.

What appears to be a perfect solution is an act of self-destruction. Sugars are absorbed quickly, so despite purging, significant amounts of calories from the binge have already been absorbed. Sugars also cause fluid retention, which can add several pounds. This is why so many bulimics either maintain or gain weight on the binge/purge cycle. Few pounds, if any, are lost.

Deadly Dangers

Persons with eating disorders may suffer the effects of severe malnutrition. They may experience such symptoms as lightheadedness, mood swings, headaches, and inability to concentrate. They may do serious damage to the digestive system, muscles, and bones as well as the functioning of major organs such as the heart.

A bulimic can wear away the enamel of her teeth and develop infection and ulcers in her esophagus from stomach acid. The most serious consequence is heart failure. The potassium lost by use of laxatives and diuretics is necessary to maintain the electrical signals that keep her body working. If the electrical messages to the heart are interrupted, she can have a heart attack.

Over-the-counter syrups that induce vomiting are dangerous. With repeated use, this poison can build up to toxic levels in the body and cause heart damage and even death. This is what happened to Karen Carpenter, the singer.

Causes of Bulimia

We live in a society that deeply fears fat. One survey stated that one-third of all women from ages nineteen to thirty-nine diet from time to time. Another survey showed that 59 percent of teenage girls today feel as if they need to lose weight.

Today's young women are products of the Weight Watchers' generation—the first generation to be raised by highly weight-conscious mothers. Many of today's teens have felt dissatisfied with their bodies as long as they can remember and have even felt their mothers were critical of their size.

Young women have learned to diet from their mothers. Their preoccupation with dieting too often seems to lead to bulimia. But bulimia is more than dieting gone haywire. This obsession with thinness is so intense that it becomes the core of a woman's identity. Thinness symbolizes strength, independence, and achievement to such women.

Many medical professionals believe bulimia is a product of modern social conflicts and lifestyle. Weak role models in parents, sexual abuse, and inability to assume adult responsibilities such as career and family have been linked to the problem.

Today women are expected to grow up to be like both their father and mother. Not only is a woman expected to be a good housekeeper and mother, but society and financial pressure often demand that she juggle a successful career, too.

The role model for women has become distorted and vague. Women fight becoming like their mothers (who do not usually work outside the home) because they fear being like them is not "enough." Many find themselves trying to fit their femaleness into some new role of maleness and femaleness that is not at all what God intended for women. Deep unhappiness is the inevitable result.

Helping the Bulimic

The bulimic, anorexic, and obese person all share a common trait—the abuse of food in an effort to cope with

the stress of everyday life. Their problem is not food but
rather an inability to face life and a sense of confusion over
who they are.

During treatment and recovery, a bulimic's hardest
physical battle is with hunger. Her hardest mental battle is
with her self-image. A bulimic is terrified of weight gain and
of eating regular meals. The starve and binge routine that
they follow distorts their appetite so that they become
conditioned to eating huge amounts of food when they
do eat.

Love and caring support are very important to the bulimic.
Most families, once they understand the problem, want to
help and be part of the solution. A good place to begin
is by talking to a family physician. Bulimia is curable.
Intensive therapy programs are available through hospitals.

New Insights on Eating Disorders

The Renfrew Center, located in Philadelphia, PA, completed a survey of more than eighty women, ages fifteen to
fifty-five who are anorexic or bulimic. Results were compared to a control group of women without eating disorders,
matched for age. The results showed the following:

1. Eighty-five percent of the women stated that prolonged
dieting is the number one factor in their eating problems.

2. Women with eating disorders begin dieting much earlier
in life than their peers. For example, 75 percent began diets
by age fifteen, as compared to 31 percent of the control
group.

3. Women with eating disorders were teased more about
their weight as they were growing up; their parents also had
problems with being overweight. Many stated that their
fathers had encouraged them to diet.

4. Fathers of many of the women with eating disorders
were alcoholics or had drinking problems.

5. By age twenty, women with eating disorders had begun self-induced vomiting and by age twenty-four had begun using laxatives.

Getting Help

Help is available. Talking to a professional who can listen and understand is important. Most people with eating disorders have spent their entire lives listening to others and trying to make them happy. The person with an eating disorder does not know how to listen to herself.

Individual therapy can help such a person learn to recognize her feelings and deal with conflicts. She can begin to feel good about who she is. She can discover positive ways to handle difficult relationships and pressures from others so that she no longer has to resort to the false security and self-destruction of food abuse.

Self-help groups are also beneficial. The support from people who are struggling with similar problems can often add insight and make food abuse sufferers feel as though they are not alone. Overeaters Anonymous is a non-profit, self-help group that is successful in helping food addicts.

Also helpful is aerobic exercise. Exercise stimulates the body to produce endorphins, which have a calming effect. Regular exercise helps keep emotions on an even keel. But even here you must be careful not to become as obsessive about exercise as you once were with food.

Gaining Control

The Renfrew Center in Philadelphia is a treatment center for bulimics and anorexics that teaches them how to regain control of their lives. Family members are brought into the sessions and trained so they will be able to help the victim when she returns to the home environment.

Honesty, courage, and willingness to change are the key ingredients to breaking free from an eating obsession.

Moderation and balance in all things are important to a sense of well-being. The food addict must focus on developing a balanced life-style. Outside interests are needed to absorb attention and bring personal satisfaction.

Taking problems to God in prayer is a wonderful way to deal with stress and to find answers. The Lord is always faithful to meet us at our point of need. Reading the Bible and other good books will bring comfort and rest to your mind and will also show you how to cope God's way. Filling your mind with good thoughts will enable you to lead a healthy, balanced life.

Not all of us receive help and healing the same way or as quickly as others. Sometimes the Lord chooses to lead us to professionals who can help us fight and win our battles. But whatever victory route He chooses for us, we know He is by our side, cheering for us, caring, guiding, and healing.

> Casting all your care upon him; for he careth for you—1 Peter 5:7, KJV.

The Lord wants you to be healthy and happy. He desires to meet us with answers at our point of need. I know of no better way to handle a problem of any kind than to cast it on the Lord.

For additional information on help for eating disorders, send a stamped, self-addressed envelope (3 stamps) plus $1.00 to the American Anorexia/Bulimia Association, 133 Cedar Lane, Teaneck, NJ 07666, (201) 836-1800. Or send $1.00 postage and handling to the National Association of Anorexia Nervosa and Associated Disorders, Box 271, Highland Park, IL 60035, (312)831-3438.

21

Little Problems with Big Names

Some health problems are not necessarily life-threatening, but they can be a nuisance that affects our well-being in many ways. You probably struggle with one or more of the "little problems" discussed in this chapter. But take heart, the answer may be simpler than you thought.

Can diet and exercise prevent or decrease our tendency toward varicose veins, hemorrhoids, TMJ, hypoglycemia, and other illnesses? Let's examine several health problems and how the way we live affects them.

Varicose Veins

Although the tendency toward varicose veins is largely hereditary, much can be done to offset their development. Exercise, diet, and support hosiery can minimize the condition that affects one in four American women and one in ten American men.

Varicose veins are more than a cosmetic problem. They also cause fatigue, pain, swelling, and cramps—not to mention the life-threatening development of phlebitis and clots. Varicose veins are much more than a nuisance.

Our lifestyles contribute to the development of varicose veins. Constipation, standing for prolonged periods of time, sitting with legs crossed, and lack of exercise will aggravate this condition.

Fiber added to the diet will relieve constipation. The varicose veins sufferer should eat plenty of vegetables and whole grains. Fresh fruits, especially citrus fruits, should be added to your diet. Scientists believe the bioflavonoids found in fruit may strengthen vein walls.

Walking, jogging, and aerobics keep the leg muscles working. Don't sit or stand still for long. Exercise keeps the blood flowing through the legs. Prop your legs up several times a day (above the heart level) to allow gravity to speed the blood flow.

Support hose also facilitates blood flow by exerting graduated pressure along the leg. Refrain from wearing tight garments such as girdles and binding belts. Don't read on the toilet. Too much pressure is placed on the leg veins in this position.

If worse comes to worse, diseased veins can be surgically removed. This procedure boasts a 96 percent cure rate. Another option is injection therapy. Diseased veins can be injected with a chemical solution, causing them to harden and wither away over a period of several months. Unfortunately, large varicose veins don't respond to this treatment. Some doctors even feel injection therapy can be dangerous.

Hemorrhoids

No one wants to admit they have hemorrhoids, but many people do. As many as eight out of ten suffer from "piles" as they are sometimes called. Most of these people are between the ages of thirty and sixty.

Many blush at discussing or admitting a hemorrhoid problem, but it is not something to be embarrassed about.

Hemorrhoids are no more than varicose veins of the rectum and anus. People can be afflicted with internal and external hemorrhoids. External hemorrhoids look like round, purple blotches, feel like soft swellings, and develop under the skin near the opening of the anus. They may cause mild to fairly severe pain.

Internal hemorrhoids are located further inside the rectum and form under the mucous membrane on the tissue lining of the rectum. Bleeding may be the only symptom associated with this condition. If internal hemorrhoids ever protrude to the outside, however, they can be extremely painful.

Pressure causes hemorrhoids—pressure from just having to stand, sit, and walk in an upright position. Constipation, pregnancy, obesity, and heavy, frequent coughing or sneezing causes hemorrhoids. People who sit a lot or lift heavy objects regularly are also more prone to hemorrhoids.

Symptoms of hemorrhoids include rectal bleeding, a feeling of fullness in the rectum at all times, and constipation.

Prevention, to a great degree, depends on cause. If constipation is the cause, then a high-fiber diet and regular exercise will help. If obesity is the cause, the obvious answer is to lose weight.

But no matter what the cause here are some tips on prevention that will work for everybody.

1. Drink lots of water—at least eight glass a day.

2. Establish regular bowel habits. Don't ever ignore the urge.

3. Exercise daily.

4. Use stool softeners with the advice of your doctor.

5. Maintain good hygiene. Just don't overdo the scrubbing of any irritated areas.

6. Avoid sugar-containing foods such as pastries, and cookies.

Have You Heard of TMJ?

In my early twenties, I suffered with TMJ disorder. The discomfort and pain were so debilitating that I suspected cancer or some other dread disease.

TMJ, short for *temporo mandibular joint* (the jaw joint in front of the ear), is a treatable problem. Symptoms include:

1. Frequent headaches in the temples, behind the eyes, in the back of the head, and like a band around the head.
2. Migraine headaches.
3. Sinus headaches.
4. Popping jaw joints when eating or yawning.
5. Stiff neck and shoulders.
6. Tingly fingers.
7. Low back pain.
8. Frequent dizziness and light-headedness.
9. Inability to open mouth very wide or even chew food.

All of this from a jaw joint that is not balanced correctly!

If you are a TMJ sufferer, neither you nor your doctor may be aware of it. You may have been sent to ear specialists, neurologists, psychiatrists, or even radiologists. Usually, no explanation for your pain can be found. You may have even been told that since no reason for your symptoms exists, you will just have to cope with the pain.

But has anyone suggested that the pain may be coming from a bad bite? TMJ is brought on by stress. Many people react to stress by tightening the muscles in their shoulders and neck and clenching their jaws.

If the jaws are clenched a lot and if the teeth are providing proper support, then the jaw joints become jammed. Overclosed jaws cause damage to the joints, resulting in a pop or crunch when the jaw is opened or closed. Arthritis can set in after many years of this. The pain adds to the stress of the sufferer and saps him of energy and strength.

The best cure for the TMJ sufferer is to relax and stop clenching his jaws. Keeping teeth apart when the mouth is closed also helps. But the answer for most people is to see a specially-trained and experienced dentist who can help in repositioning the lower jaw.

Poor eating habits can also contribute to TMJ by adding to internal stress. Your dentist will no doubt insist on dietary changes if this is your problem.

Relief for this painful condition came when I started eating a balanced diet, exercising regularly, and found mental and spiritual healing.

Night Blindness

An early sign of vitamin A deficiency is the difficulty in adjusting to seeing in darkness.

Under normal conditions, our eyes can adjust to darkness in a matter of seconds. When fifteen to twenty minutes are required to make the adjustment, the problem is diagnosed as night blindness.

Vitamin A supplementation will help improve night vision. Good sources of vitamin A include sweet potatoes, carrots, spinach, cantaloupe, broccoli, winter squash, and apricots.

What Did You Say?

Elevated blood cholesterol, high blood pressure, excessive caffeine, and too many cigarettes can limit blood flow through the tiny artery in each inner ear and can lead to hearing loss.

Research conducted twenty-five years ago showed that a low-fat diet not only benefits the heart but the hearing as well. To assure good hearing, drop whole milk from your diet and substitute skim milk. Your ear bones need the vitamin D and calcium found in skim milk.

Other nutrients needed by the ear include beta-carotene, vitamin A, and zinc. Research has linked zinc supplements to a marked improvement in hearing. Just remember, any vitamin supplementation must be under a doctor's guidance.

Putting Dizziness on a Diet

If neither you nor your doctor can provide an explanation for your chronic dizziness, take a look at your diet. You may be eating yourself into a case of vertigo.

In a study of one hundred patients who suffered from dizziness, hearing loss and/or ringing in the ears, many of them were overweight and had high cholesterol and triglyceride levels in their blood. Some were insulin resistant, which meant their cells had trouble using insulin even when there were normal amounts in the blood. Only 4 percent of these patients had low blood sugar showing that hypoglycemia may be overrated as a cause of vertigo.

When the patients were put on calorie-cutting, low-fat, low-sugar diets, their dizziness disappeared in most cases. The dietary treatment for dizziness would also be helpful in preventing heart disease.

Hypoglycemia

Hypoglycemia is an abnormally low concentration of sugar in the blood. One of the best ways to treat hypoglycemia is through a strict diet. Avoid sugars such as jellies, honey, sugar, candies, cookies, pies, cakes, and sweetened carbonated beverages.

Complex carbohydrates can be eaten by the person with hypoglycemia because current research indicates that starch meals result in significantly lower plasma glucose and insulin levels in the body.

Small, frequent feedings help prevent fluctuations in blood glucose levels with time spans of no greater than five hours between meals. A good snack would include a complex carbohydrate and a protein source. Avoid alcoholic beverages altogether.

In the past doctors recommended a high protein, low carbohydrate diet for sufferers of hypoglycemia. New evidence suggests that mixed meals of complex carbohydrates will relieve symptoms without subjecting the patient to the complications that often result from a low-carbohydrate diet.

Diabetes

Five to six million Americans have diabetes. Many have it and don't even know it. Almost all diabetes is inherited but almost all can be controlled if caught early.

There are two kinds of diabetes: *Type I or juvenile onset diabetes* and *Type II or adult onset diabetes.* Both lead to a lack of insulin, which helps burn excess blood sugar.

Type I diabetes requires daily injections of insulin. Type II diabetes can be treated with diet and drugs. Because Type II diabetics are prone to obesity, weight loss is often all that is needed to control their disease.

Type II diabetes involves inadequate use of insulin. Cells have receptors on their surfaces that normally respond to insulin. But when insulin attaches to the receptors, the cells take up sugar from the blood. If the cells don't have enough insulin receptors, the sugar stays in the bloodstream and diabetes results.

Tests have shown that a diet high in complex carbohydrates can help diabetics bring down blood sugar levels. Exercise makes the cells more sensitive to insulin by increasing the number of insulin receptors.

Type II diabetics may be four times more susceptible to heart disease than non-diabetics. The same diet that helps diabetics will help those prone to heart disease.

Foods that Help

Some good news for the diabetic was recently announced. For the first time in ten years, the "Exchange Lists for Meal Planning," which are used by diabetics to control blood sugar, were revised and expanded. The starch-bread group has replaced the meat group as number one on the list. The American Diabetes Association is now emphasizing the benefits of starchy foods (complex carbohydrates) such as whole-grain breads, cereals, and rice.

In fact, the new list encourages people to consume 50 to 60 percent of their calories from carbohydrates. The old list recommended 45 percent carbohydrates. To compensate for the added carbohydrate calories, reduce fat intake. New recommendations are to lower daily fat intake from 35 to 30 percent.

Fiber and Diabetes

Foods high in fiber also help the diabetic by slowing down the release of sugar into the bloodstream. This prevents a sudden demand for insulin, which is responsible for guiding sugar molecules to the cells to be burned for fuel.

Since nearly half of all diabetics are overweight, fiber comes in handy in weight loss. Fiber fills you up, not out, and satisfies the appetite while adding few calories. Studies have proven that people will lose weight when they eat a high fiber diet.

Diabetics no longer have to resign themselves to a life of chronic obesity and daily insulin injections. Some doctors are now recommending high-fiber diets to reduce weight and insulin needs.

One physician stated he was able to reduce the insulin needs of his patients by as much as 25 to 100 percent depending on the type diabetes. The people who discontinued using insulin are those who would not have needed insulin at all had they been eating right.

Most recent research is showing that by supplementing the diet of non-insulin-dependent diabetics with omega-3 fatty acids, the patient's sensitivity to his own insulin can be heightened. Fish oil, which contains omega-3 fatty acids, seems to improve the effectiveness of insulin.

The pancreas of the non-insulin dependent diabetic produces insulin in amounts that vary from too little to too much to normal. These people have usually developed the disease because of obesity, and they tend to be resistant to insulin.

Fruit and Insulin Levels

Fresh fruit is an excellent food for diabetics. This natural source of fiber is low in calories, salt, and fat and is rich in vitamins and minerals.

Fresh fruits contain the natural sugars that give energy without too rapid a rise in blood sugar levels. When fruit reaches the stomach, passage of the meal into the intestine is slowed. A gel-like fiber such as pectin, which is found in apples and citrus fruits, coats the intestinal lining. This protective coating slows the absorption of glucose. Keeping glucose in check is important because wild swings in glucose levels cause insulin levels to react similarly.

Researchers studied insulin levels after volunteers consumed different forms of the same food. Studies showed that insulin levels jumped dramatically after drinking orange juice, but rose slowly after eating whole oranges.

Scientists say this happens because the fiber in apples and oranges helps keep glucose and insulin levels from changing rapidly. Fruit fiber also leaves you feeling full longer than most foods and, therefore, aids in weight loss. This is why vitamins can never be a substitute for fresh fruit. Fruit is really a healing food.

Three Steps to Health

The logo of the American Diabetes Association is a triangle divided into three parts:
1. One is for diet.
2. Another is for insulin.
3. The other is for exercise.

Most diabetics know their life depends on controlling blood sugar, weight, and blood pressure. Exercise helps in all three of these areas.

A diabetic should exercise only with a doctor's guidance. Doing too much too fast can be dangerous for them. For many diabetics, a diet and exercise program are all they need in order to control the disease.

Those who suffer from illnesses as varied as chronic dizziness and varicose veins may find help in that same combination of diet and exercise. Medical research reveals that most people have more say in their health than previously thought. Make some quality decisions regarding your own eating and exercising habits. You'll be glad you did!

—————22—————
Bringing Down Your Blood Pressure

I recently read a magazine article that was based on the celebration of a man's fifty-ninth birthday. What's so unusual about that? The man's father had died at age forty-four, obese and hooked on three packs of cigarettes a day. This man was celebrating that through proper diet, exercise, and no smoking, he had beat the odds of dying an early death.

Many factors contribute to heart disease, but high blood pressure, cigarette smoking, and elevated blood cholesterol levels are at the top of the list. All three of these factors are within our control to some degree through modifying our lifestyles. Other important factors include male gender, obesity, gout, diabetes, inactivity, stress, and inherited tendencies toward the disease.

In this chapter we will focus on the effects of high blood pressure and smoking. Because high cholesterol levels are more complicated to understand and detect, we will devote an entire chapter to this silent killer.

Crash Dieting and Blood Pressure

Since many of you reading this book are on a diet or are thinking of dieting, let me warn you once again that crash dieting and yo-yo dieting (fasting and feasting) can not only bring on high blood pressure but heart failure as well. Overweight people are twice as likely to have hypertension as normal weight people. The evidence points to the dieting patterns of the overweight person as being their biggest health problem.

High blood pressure occurs when the brain produces a potent stress hormone. This same hormone is triggered when one is frightened. The brain signals danger, and this stress hormone causes the heartbeat to increase, blood vessels to constrict, and blood pressure to rise.

A severe reduction in calorie intake, like that associated with a crash diet, will trigger the production of this hormone. Overeating is stressful and can cause the brain to signal production of the hormone. The body seems to have a natural system of linking blood pressure and caloric intake.

The best way to break out of the hypertension cycle is to exercise, eat a sensible diet, and avoid crash dieting. Physical activity can reset the systems that control metabolism and weight regulation. Exercise lowers blood pressure by slowing the production of the stress hormone and strengthening the heart.

Crash dieting only makes a person fatter, weaker, and sicker. In contrast, a gradual weight loss through exercise and a safe, balanced diet will protect your blood pressure and give more lasting results.

Put Your Heart into Losing Weight

Did you know that when your body loses weight, your heart does also? When you have an overweight heart, the risk of death is twice as high with people who already have high blood pressure.

When you are overweight your body calls for a greater flow of blood for fuel. But instead of pumping blood faster, it pumps more blood with each beat. This makes the heart begin to build up extra tissue to help it push harder.

The heart of an obese person can build up so much tissue that it becomes enlarged and musclebound. Because obesity usually leads to hypertension and high blood pressure, you have a formula for real trouble. The increased heart mass can cause arrhythmias or irregular beating of the heart that can, in extreme cases, lead to sudden death.

A safe diet can reduce body weight, blood pressure, and the size of the heart. A three-year study of forty-one overweight patients who had high blood pressure showed that losing weight with a safe diet reduced blood pressure and size of the heart.

The forty-one patients were divided into three groups. One group was put on a safe, balanced diet recommended by the American Heart Association. Another group was put on a medication to reduce blood pressure, and the other group was placed on a placebo. Heart sizes were checked at the beginning and end of the test.

In the end, the dieting patients lost an average of 18 pounds in twenty-one weeks. Blood pressures fell to normal, and heart size was reduced. There were no significant changes in heart size with the other two groups.

If you are overweight with high blood pressure, take the medication your doctor prescribes and also pursue a safe, balanced diet. If you are obese but do not yet have high blood pressure, chances are pretty good that you will develop it, especially if you are a post-menopausal woman. Avoid high-protein and crash diets that will deplete the heart of potassium and magnesium and increase irregularity of heart beats.

Salt and High Blood Pressure

Never think you cannot do without salt. Research has shown that the less salt you use, the less you will want. Craving for salt comes from overuse. Craving salt never reflects a need of the body but a habit or an addiction.

Some blood pressure drugs actually cause a person to crave salty foods. By reducing the amount of sodium in the body, the drugs trigger the body to call for more salt. This becomes a dangerous situation because if a patient eats more salt, the doctor will think the diuretics are not working. He will then increase the dosage or even add new drugs, and the patient ends up in worse shape.

If you are on medication for blood pressure, it is essential that you follow a reduced-salt diet. Remember the more salt you eat, the more you will want. If you stick with a low-salt routine for two or three months, you'll actually prefer less salt.

Fresh fruit has little if any sodium and is ideal for people with a tendency to high blood pressure. Fruits with potassium are especially beneficial. Researchers have found that a high-potassium diet, like that followed by vegetarians, leads to lower incidence of high blood pressure. Potassium can be found in such fruits as bananas, cantaloupes, and apricots.

Controlling High Blood Pressure

New studies have shown the possibility of lowering high blood pressure without drugs. Using lifestyle changes in areas of relaxation, diet, and exercise, researchers have helped high blood pressure (HBP) sufferers lower their numbers. For those who are borderline or mildly hypertensive, several behavior techniques should be tried before resorting to medication.

One is relaxation. All doctors agree that blood pressure is affected by mental stress. Research has shown that sufferers of hypertension are able to maintain normal blood pressure and stay off medication after learning relaxation techniques such as breathing slowly and deeply or warming hands and feet to relax muscles.

Another way to keep blood pressure down is through diet and the control of salt intake. Studies have also shown that combining coffee and cigarettes will significantly elevate the blood pressure.

A large intake of alcohol can also cause high blood pressure. Studies show that women drinking only two mixed drinks a day were 40 percent more likely to develop high blood pressure than non-drinkers.

The same study showed that women who drank the equivalent of three glasses of milk decreased their risk of high blood pressure by 22 percent. I hope you choose skim milk over whole or 2 percent milk because of its low fat content. Just skip the alcohol for your health's sake.

How to Lower Your Blood Pressure

Aerobic exercise is helpful in lowering blood pressure by making the heart more efficient and by assisting the body in handling stress. When the heart beats more efficiently, the heart rate is reduced. Many times I have heard it said that "exercise is nature's best tranquilizer."

Studies have shown that regular aerobic exercise such as brisk walking, jogging, swimming, and biking produces moderate reductions in blood pressure in people with mild to moderate hypertension. (Weight lifting is not recommended because it can actually raise blood pressure.)

In some cases, physicians have been able to reduce or discontinue HBP medications entirely through a carefully monitored exercise program. The only drawback is that once off the exercise program the high blood pressure will return to its former level.

Communicating with Your Heart

Did you know that the blood pressures of spouses are similar and become even more so the longer two people are married? Even when other risk factors are taken into account, the blood pressure of spouses seem to remain similar.

This similarity may come from the way couples deal with conflict and express their emotions.

Medical scientists believe that we not only communicate with words but with our entire bodies, including our hearts and cardiovascular systems. Human communication is the greatest factor that influences blood pressure. Maybe that's why the Bible repeatedly warns that life and death are in the power of the tongue.

> Pleasant words are a honeycomb, sweet to the soul and healing to the bones—Proverbs 16:24, NIV.

> Reckless words pierce like a sword, but the tongue of the wise brings healing—Proverbs 12:18, NIV.

Did you know that talking boosts your blood pressure and listening lowers it? Many people suffering with high blood pressure talk too fast and do not listen when others speak. When they do listen, they listen "on guard," anxiously waiting for a chance to be heard again.

There are ways to combat these personality traits that contribute to high blood pressure. Tests show that when sufferers of HBP learned to speak more slowly and breathe regularly during conversation, their blood pressures stayed more in the normal range.

Learning to be a relaxed listener can also help. Talking itself does not raise blood pressure, but the emotions behind the talking do. Even deaf people with HBP problems suffer from similar symptoms when they're engaged in animated communication with hand signs. One study noted that blood pressure rose when people were asked to "speed" read as opposed to normal reading.

Studies show that paying calm attention to some activity outside of yourself brings blood pressure down. Caring for a pet can be very relaxing. Doing a favor for someone may do more good for you than for them!

Listening instead of fighting to be heard can be therapeutic and can keep you out of trouble. Talking is for adults what crying is for a baby—an avenue to express your problems and needs. But when these needs go unfulfilled, the talking creates problems and stress.

My advice? Pour out your problems before the Lord and leave them there with Him. He longs to take our burdens and bear them for us. He tells us that through our weaknesses, He can be strong. He wants us to rest and relax in Him. Realizing that an all-knowing God still loves and accepts us, we do not have to be overly concerned about what others think of us. Unshakable faith in Christ allows us to relax more and not feel threatened by others.

Picture a clear, beautiful blue pool of peaceful water in the very center of your being. Imagine yourself surrounded by shade trees and the quiet of a forest. With the Lord's help, you can feel just that peaceful on the inside. Learn to operate from that peaceful place of rest in Jesus.

Jesus said, "Come to me, all you who are weary and burdened, and I will give you rest" (Matthew 11:28, NIV).

But What About Heredity?

The knowledge that heart disease runs in your family can be used to your advantage. Sure, genes have a lot to do with how long you live. But with proper diet and exercise, you can lower the risk of that disease attacking you.

By now it should be pretty clear that exercise can prolong your life. One authority has estimated that for every hour of exercise, you can live an extra two hours.

Other studies have shown that a minimum of three hours of exercise weekly will expend at least 2,000 calories and will decrease the chance of heart attack by one-third. Not only will you add years to your life with exercise, you will add life to your years.

Your genes and your lifestyle are intertwined in ways that scientists are just beginning to understand. There is a big difference between genetic disorder and genetic tendency toward disease. A *genetic disorder* means you carry a disease in your genes that is beyond your control. A *genetic tendency* means you have inherited a predisposition to a certain disease.

Though you may carry the risk of having a heart attack, for example, your fate is not sealed. Your environment will have a lot to do with whether or not you have the disease. There are many ways to offset a genetic trend. Often what is inherited is not the disease itself but a weakness or condition that can lead to the disease.

Warning Signs of Heart Disease

Knowing the symptoms of a heart attack can save your life or the life of someone else. The American Heart Association reports that thousands of people die each year because they did not know the warning signs of a heart attack. Here are the symptoms:

1. Uncomfortable pressure, fullness, squeezing, or pain in the center of the chest, lasting two minutes or more.
2. Pain in shoulders, neck, and arm.
3. Severe pain, dizziness, fainting, sweating, nausea, or shortness of breath.

The following actions should be taken when symptoms occur:

1. Stop what you are doing and sit or lie down.
2. Act at once if pain lasts for two minutes or more by calling the emergency medical service or have someone take you to an emergency room.

If you think you are having a heart attack, don't wait. Call for help immediately.

Stroke and High Blood Pressure

Stroke is the death of brain cells after a blood vessel that carries oxygen to the brain bursts or is blocked with a clot. Stroke victims are left with paralysis of the muscles controlled by the half of the brain that was stricken. Strokes cause an estimated 155,000 deaths in America each year.

Stroke, once viewed as a single, life-shattering trauma, is now seen as a treatable circulation disease. As one neurosurgeon put it, stroke is now viewed as the brain's version of a heart attack. Like heart attacks, strokes can be prevented.

High blood pressure, which is linked to half of all strokes, is now treatable. Some clots that formerly blocked blood vessels and caused strokes can be dissolved; the formation of new ones can even be prevented. Medical science has learned how to re-open clogged arteries with tiny balloons and lasers. Blockages can be by-passed in some cases. Blood can be thickened or thinned as needed.

Stroke Prevention

Experiments on enriching the spinal fluid also show promise for the stroke victim. Laboratory experiments with animals left brain-dead by strokes have had surprising results. These animals were revived to full function by a technique that enriched the spinal fluid with oxygen. Although nothing has been done to test this on humans, researchers are exploring this method as a possible treatment for stroke victims.

Diet also plays a role in stroke prevention. Researchers have found that eating lots of fruits and vegetables gives the body added potassium, which may prevent strokes. In fact, just one extra serving of fruits or vegetables each day may decrease the risk of stroke by as much as 40 percent!

A banana a day just may keep stroke away. Research with 859 adults over twelve years showed that those with plenty of potassium in their diets were 40 percent less likely to suffer a fatal stroke.

Scientists believe that potassium enables the brain to survive a lack of oxygen longer, lessening the damage of a potential stroke. All the facts are not in yet, but it seems an excellent idea to eat potassium-rich vegetables and fruits, doesn't it?

Smoking and Heart Disease

Studies have shown that cigarette smoking doubles the risk of heart attack in the general population. For those who have a family history of heart disease, it increases the risk four times.

Smoking affects the heart by giving conflicting signals. Nicotine simultaneously tells the muscles to relax and yet speeds up the cardiovascular system.

Cigarette smoking adversely affects cholesterol levels. A study of teens who smoked an average of three cigarettes a day showed they were experiencing high cholesterol and triglyceride levels. The more they smoked, the higher the levels in their bodies.

Recent research has shown a new risk factor that may contribute to heart disease—a high white blood cell count (WBC). People with a high white blood cell count seem to have a greater chance of developing heart disease. White blood cells normally increase in number to fight infection, but if their count remains high, they can cause damage to artery walls and eventual atherosclerosis.

A fairly recent study also indicates that cigarette smoke causes "killer cells," or those cells that help destroy tumors in the body, to be impotent and useless.

Although smoking is not the only cause of a high white blood cell count, it definitely seems to be a factor. When individuals with a high white blood cell count quit smoking, their count dropped sharply. Smokers with a high white blood cell count are extremely vulnerable to heart attack.

Smoking and Your Life Span

Every smoker will eventually destroy his lungs. Irreparable damage is not a possibility; it is a certainty, unless emphysema chokes him to death first. A heart attack or cancer of the lungs, throat, voice box, or bladder can even finish the job sooner.

Smokers have a 2,500 times greater risk of developing lung cancer than nonsmokers. On the average, non-smokers will outlive smokers by at least two years. In the case of a family with predisposition to heart disease, a non-smoker will outlive the smoker by ten to fifteen years.

Smokers are sick more often than non-smokers and are more easily infected with germs and viruses. Some businesses try to avoid hiring smokers because of their higher absenteeism rate. Their secondary cigarette smoke also poses a health risk to nonsmoking employees.

Cigarettes are the most common and costly drug addiction because smoking is linked to so many other diseases. Heart attack, cancer, and emphysema are aggravated by the use of nicotine. For all the harm caused by cigarettes, it's a wonder that the tobacco industry is allowed to continue to advertise this "drug" to young and old.

Kicking the Habit

There are many ways to stop smoking. People who are desperate to break their nicotine addiction have tried everything from using filters that gradually decrease the smoke they inhale to dipping their cigarettes in vinegar. Others replace smoking cigarettes with chewing carrots or celery. Everyone seems to have a gimmick that guarantees success.

Many people have found that a fifteen-minute walk helps beat the urge to smoke. Others have found deep breathing to be effective because taking deep breaths mimics the action of inhaling tobacco smoke without the damage. The best way to stop smoking is to realize what you're doing to your body and just quit. Sadly, however, quitting "cold turkey" seems impossible for most people because they are hooked.

Those who just can't seem to quit often try to compromise by switching to cigars, pipes, or chewing tobacco. The risk of lip and mouth cancer is still great with these alternatives. Don't assume that low-tar and low-nicotine cigarettes are the answer, either. They are no safer than regular cigarettes.

Smokers are used to a certain degree of satisfaction from a cigarette. With a low-tar, low-nicotine cigarette smokers must puff longer and inhale deeper to achieve the same satisfaction. Studies of the nicotine content in the blood after smoking have shown that those who smoke the so-called safer cigarettes have the same concentration of nicotine as those who smoke the regular cigarettes.

Why People Smoke

Through diet and exercise one woman had been able to turn her life around, take years off her face, and give up smoking. But resisting the urge to smoke was much more difficult each time she drank a cup of coffee.

Her addiction to smoking was much harder to break than her bad eating habits because she had both a physical and mental addiction to cigarettes. Most people can break a physical addiction in two or three weeks, but taming a psychological addiction can take much longer.

Smoking is learned behavior that gives a person instant satisfaction. When cigarettes are combined with coffee or alcohol, the temporary, pleasurable feelings become intertwined. When you indulge in one, you automatically crave the other. That's why drinking coffee always brought on the need for a cigarette in this lady.

Those who are serious about kicking the habit must avoid the coffee, for example, and substitute juice or water. Learn why you smoke. Is it out of boredom, frustration, or for the lift? Exercise can generate the same benefits as a cigarette, and simultaneously improve your health instead of destroying it. Change daily patterns so that the void left by cigarettes will be filled with less harmful activities.

Consider the Consequences

Focusing on the bad aspects of smoking also helps curb the urge. Remind yourself what nicotine does to your lungs. Remember the dull taste buds, the burning throat, the nausea. When you consider the consequences, smoking is so foolish. Why do it?

One of the most unattractive things a woman can do is smoke. Smoking used to be considered glamorous when all the big movie stars smoked. Women are finally realizing that smoking ages their skin, gives them bad breath, decreases lung capacity, stains their teeth, and causes them to reek of stale tobacco. If the health risks involved with smoking are not a deterrent, the beauty risks should count for something.

Smoking can harm those around you—your children, your co-workers, and your spouse. The effects are seen most clearly in children whose parents smoke. These youngsters show increased instances of ear infections; decreased airway function; increased need for tonsillectomies and adenoidectomies; increased incidence of lower-respiratory tract infections; and elevated overall risk of cancer.

Tobacco smoke makes a significant contribution to indoor air pollution. Breathing secondary smoke can cause sinus discomfort, eye irritation, coughing, and sneezing. No one should be exposed to another's smoke.

Gaining Weight or Losing Your Life

"Fear of fat" is the most common excuse given by female smokers when asked why they won't quit. Research has shown that ex-smokers seem to develop a sweet tooth.

Giving in to that urge will add calories and pile on the pounds. When you come off nicotine, you are not doomed to gain weight. You may want to eat more, however, so go for carrots, celery, and fruits.

Some experts say when you quit smoking your metabolism slows down. Although this has not been proven by scientists, you would be wise to increase your activity level when you quit smoking to avoid possible weight gain. A brisk, thirty-minute walk will burn 210 calories and boost your metabolism for a while. Exercise will also give you a physical and mental boost that beats a nicotine high.

Even if you should gain a few extra pounds, the benefits of removing a known carcinogen like nicotine from your life will do wonders for your health.

High blood pressure and smoking, two major contributors to heart disease, can be controlled to some degree. If you smoke, quit immediately. Others have done it, and you can, too. If you don't smoke, avoid that life-threatening vice by never starting. High blood pressure sufferers can lower their reading by learning to relax, exercising, losing weight, and eating a low-fat, low-salt diet. Good health is not primarily the result of pre-determined, hereditary factors but a series of wise, daily choices that anyone can make.

—23—

You Can Lower Your Cholesterol Level

The National Cholesterol Education Program (NCEP) reports that 75 percent of Americans know that high blood cholesterol leads to heart attack. Yet only 46 percent have ever had their blood cholesterol checked, and fewer than 5 percent know what their cholesterol levels actually are.

The only difference between people, particularly men, who die at age 40 with clogged arteries as opposed to those who die after 70 with the same, is the rate at which their arteries become clogged.

What Is Cholesterol?

Cholesterol is a form of fat that circulates in the blood. Despite its bad reputation, cholesterol strengthens cell walls, produces cell membranes, and is essential to good health.

Cholesterol is also a necessary part of many hormones, including the sex hormones testosterone and estrogen, and other hormones made by the testes, ovaries, and adrenal glands. All the cholesterol your body requires can be made by the liver. Too much cholesterol is dangerous, but the body cells must have some cholesterol in order to function.

In order to travel in the bloodstream, cholesterol hitches a ride on special proteins call lipoproteins. Lipoproteins make cholesterol soluble and keep it from clumping up in the arteries. Two major forms of lipoproteins are high-density lipoproteins (HDL) and low-density proteins (LDL). The LDL cholesterol tends to pile up in the arteries and causes heart attacks.

Special receptors on cells bind to the protein cholesterol and bring it into a cell. People who inherit a cholesterol problem have only half the normal number of these receptors, which decreases the ability of the cells to absorb cholesterol from the blood. When cholesterol cannot get into the cells as quickly as it should, it keeps circulating in the bloodstream. The longer cholesterol stays in circulation, the longer it has time to pile up on artery walls.

Keep It Moving

Studies have shown that HDL cholesterol actually lowers the risk of heart attack. This cholesterol is not deposited in the arteries. Instead, it is sent to the liver where it is changed into bile salts and eventually travels to the digestive tract. In the form of bile salts, the cholesterol helps convert food fats for digestion.

Medicine is now available that will help take the cholesterol safely out of the bloodstream. Eating certain foods will also aid in removing cholesterol from the bloodstream. A low-fat diet will eventually slow down the clogging process.

Triglycerides are another form of fat that circulates in the blood besides cholesterol. Both of these fats are essential to health, and both are necessary to the bloodstream. Excessive amounts, however, can be lethal.

Triglycerides are the burning fats used for energy or fuel. They are stored all over the body just under the skin as fat. They come from the liver and the diet. After digestion, fats from food float in the blood for one or two hours before being taken out of the blood by fat tissue called lipoproteins. If the fat is not removed correctly from the blood, then fat intake must be restricted to prevent build-up in the blood and arteries.

Lifestyle or Heredity?

Most heart disease starts in your stomach. Back in the 1950s, scientific tests proved that healthy young volunteers who were fed butter experienced increased blood cholesterol levels. Soon a cause and effect relationship was pieced together that showed coronary artery disease, which now kills 40 percent of adult Americans, is a nutritional disorder. Bypass surgery is increasingly considered to be an insufficient answer.

If heart disease runs in your family, chances are the genes that regulate fatty substances in the blood may be involved. By keeping your weight down, exercising regularly, cutting fat intake, eating foods rich in polyunsaturates (such as fish and chicken), shunning red meats, and lowering salt intake, you can greatly reduce any risk of heart attack.

Medicines are also available to aid you in handling the fat in your bloodstream. Although your body's response to your diet is regulated to a degree by hereditary factors, the nutrient content of your food is critical to the condition of your arteries.

Detecting the Silent Killer

If you have a broken leg or hives, you know something is obviously wrong and you seek a doctor. Detecting heart disease, however, is not so simple. Cholesterol can silently build up in your arteries over the years, narrow the arteries, and slow the blood flow to a trickle. A heart attack can strike without warning. In many cases, heart attack victims experienced no hint of trouble beforehand.

This is why it's so important to have your cholesterol checked. Children as well as adults should be tested each year for cholesterol levels. Prevention is always so much better than treatment. Doctors can peek into your arteries, so to speak, and see what is happening. People may not like physicals, but proper testing is like a sneak preview that allows you to avoid a bad movie.

To find out if you have cholesterol build-up, ask your doctor to conduct the necessary tests at a time in your life when your diet is not changing and you are not gaining or losing weight. For a cholesterol check, blood can be taken on the spot. You must fast overnight, however, for an accurate triglyceride check.

Your cholesterol reading will vary just as your blood pressure and weight varies. If your cholesterol count is over 200, further tests should be made, especially if there is a family history of heart disease. The ideal count would be 180 or below.

If your cholesterol reading is high, the first thing you should do is change your diet. Your doctor will give you a list of foods to eat, probably the diet recommended by the American Heart Association. This diet is low in fat and high in fiber foods like fruits, vegetables, and whole grains.

Don't expect overnight results. Learning new eating habits may take time. Once you settle into a low-fat diet like that of the American Heart Association, you will begin to see a change for the better in your cholesterol levels.

Planning a Healthy Diet

Plan a diet that will work for you. Blood levels of cholesterol can be decreased by reducing meat intake, egg yolks, and butter fat. One diet that works well divides each day's calories into 20 percent protein, 20 percent fat, and 60 percent fiber-rich complex carbohydrates such as grains, beans, fruits, vegetables, and nuts.

Everyone should reduce fat intake by reducing and entirely cutting such foods as butter, whole milk and whole milk cheeses, ice cream, hotdogs, hamburgers, sausage, and lunch meat. Forget about egg yolks and organ meats on any kind of regular basis.

A major contributor to high cholesterol is saturated fats. These fats are usually hard at room temperature and are found in meats, dairy products, and foods fried in lard, shortening, palm, or coconut oil.

On the other hand, polyunsaturates are soft or liquid at room temperature and are found mostly in vegetable oils such as safflower, sunflower, corn, soybean, and cottonseed. These fats help decrease the bad cholesterol in the blood. In fact, studies indicate that monounsaturated fats, such as olive and peanut oils, may be even more effective in decreasing total cholesterol levels.

Saturated fats from beef, pork, and other livestock as well as cooking oils made from corn and soybeans contain what biochemists call omega-6 fatty acids. Omega-6 fatty acids are associated with heart disease and colon, prostate, and breast cancer.

Heavy intake of omega-6 fats cause excessive production of hormone-like materials that seem to trigger the formation of tumors and the development of atherosclerosis in the arteries (or the slow build-up of artery-wall fats often responsible for choking off blood flow to the heart).

Once you get your cholesterol down to a safe level, you can indulge occasionally in a favorite food from the high-cholesterol list, but basically you need to remain on the diet described above in order to maintain acceptable cholesterol levels. Changing your diet is much better than drug therapy in combating cholesterol.

The American Heart Association offers the following recommendations for a healthy heart:

1. Reduce total fat intake to 25 to 30 percent of your daily calorie intake.

2. Increase intake of carbohydrates such as grains, and beans

3. Maintain a desirable weight.

4. Reduce dietary cholesterol.

Fighting Cholesterol with Fiber

Adding fiber to the diet will help in the fight against cholesterol. Fiber comes in two forms: water-soluble and water-insoluble. *Water-insoluble fibers,* like those found in wheat products, aid in digestion and elimination and help reduce the risk of colon cancer. *Water-soluble fibers* are also good for your digestion, but they have the added benefit of forming a gel around cholesterol molecules that keeps them from being absorbed into the bloodstream. This prevents build-up and clogging of the arteries.

For example, the pectin in fruit is thought to help prevent heart disease. Researchers believe pectin captures excess cholesterol in the digestive tract and flushes it out of the body before it can be reabsorbed. Pectin may also help to raise the level of good cholesterol in the bloodstream.

Fiber works very quickly in lowering cholesterol levels. Some patients experience as much as a 20 percent reduction in cholesterol in as little as eleven days when two fiber sources, like oats and fruit, were added to their diets. No other changes were needed in their diets to accomplish these amazing results.

Recent experiments that place people on diets rich in water-soluble fibers have been successful in lowering cholesterol and other blood fats. Good sources of water-soluble fibers include: oat bran, oatmeal, dried beans, fruit (with peeling), and raw vegetables.

Foods that Lower Cholesterol

We have already seen that skim milk lowers cholesterol. There are other foods that also seem to work the same magic.

Fiber in oats has long been known to lower blood cholesterol in people with extremely high levels. Studies have shown that just two ounces of oatmeal a day can lower cholesterol by almost 5 percent within a few weeks. Even less amounts than this can mean an improvement in the blood cholesterol. Some doctors say the cholesterol-lowering ability of oats is as effective as the drugs for the disease.

What in oats brings about these miraculous changes? Soluble fiber forms a gel as it moves through the intestines, and in some ways not fully understood, interferes with the absorption or metabolism of cholesterol.

Don't expect oats to work wonders for you if you maintain a high-fat, high-cholesterol diet. If you really want to attack cholesterol, eat more than two ounces of oatmeal or oat bran each day. Just remember to include other necessary carbohydrates in your diet.

Other foods that fight cholesterol include beans and fish. Researchers believe fiber is the part of beans that does the job on cholesterol.

Carrots and Cholesterol

If you're fighting cholesterol, you want carrots in your diet. They contain calcium pectate, a substance that is thought to lower blood cholesterol. Onions, broccoli, and cabbage also contain this substance.

In one study healthy volunteers were given seven ounces of carrots, or about two medium ones, a day for three weeks. Their blood cholesterol levels were lowered by 11 percent.

Studies by the USDA indicate that the cholesterol-lowering agent is located in the fiber of the carrot and is called calcium pectate. What seems to happen is that the calcium pectate binds with bile acids. Since cholesterol is needed to make bile acids in the liver, less cholesterol goes to the blood when calcium pectate is present.

The pectin fiber in fruits like apples and grapefruit also lowers cholesterol, though less than carrots. Fiber from oats and beans does an even better job.

A well-balanced diet that includes lots of fresh vegetables and fruits should help lower your cholesterol. A nice addition to the package deal will be the lost weight on such a diet. Carrot fiber is a great filler and has no calories.

Cold Water Fish

Salmon and many other fish such as cod, herring, sardines, anchovies, and mackerel contain EPA (eicosapentaenoic acid), which causes cholesterol to drop. Another good source of EPA would be two teaspoons of cod-liver oil a day.

A diet rich in ocean fish oil also markedly reduces triglycerides in the blood by reducing its manufacture by the liver.

Research on Eskimos in Greenland led to the discovery that eating fish lowers cholesterol. These Eskimos eat a diet high in fat and cholesterol, yet they suffer no heart disease. Why? It's the cold water fish they eat. The coldness of the water seems to be the key factor.

Cholesterol is directly tied to saturated fats. Saturated fats are solid at room temperature. Examples are lard and vegetable shortenings. Saturated fats are the villains in heart disease.

On the other hand, unsaturated fats actually reduce cholesterol, lower triglyceride levels, and help prevent blood clots from forming. Fish oil is highly unsaturated, almost twice as unsaturated as any vegetable oil. The colder the water, the more unsaturated the oils have to be to stay in a fluid state within the fish. Therefore, fish from cold water are the best.

Omega-3 Fatty Acids

Highly-unsaturated fats are called omega-3 fatty acids. They lower cholesterol, thin the blood, and make platelets less sticky by becoming infused in the red blood cell membranes. Although the process is not completely understood, omega-3s somehow sweep cholesterol out of the blood.

Fish oils change the delicate balance of blood components called lipoproteins that carry cholesterol around the body. Omega-3s force down the levels of lipoproteins that carry cholesterol and triglycerides into body tissues and push up the level of HDLs, a lipoprotein that carries cholesterol away to be discarded.

Is fish really brain food? Yes, research indicates that omega-3s are a prominent part of gray matter. Studies have also shown that depriving young animals of omega-3s during the periods in which their brains are still growing can impair visual and mental functioning. So how important are omega-3s to human brain development? Researchers believe they are vital to mother and baby.

Farm-fed fish will not lower your cholesterol like cold-water fish will. They have been fed soybean meal. Frying fish in vegetable oil destroys the effects of omega-3s. Baking or broiling fish is best.

What are the best sources of omega-3s? These valuable unsaturated fats can be found in salmon (canned or fresh), mackerel, American eel, herring, rainbow trout, lake whitefish, oysters, and squid.

Doctors and researchers recommend that you eat all the fresh-water fish you can and maintain a balanced diet. The omega-3s consumed in eating one-third to one-half pound of fresh salmon per day are enough to create heart-benefiting changes in the blood. But who can afford that or even get that much down?

Nutritionists suggest a once-a-week-meal of omega-3-rich fish. If you can eat more than that, great! Americans still only eat 12 or 13 pounds of fish and shellfish each year compared to 165 pounds of red meat.

Sardines seem to contain the highest percentage of omega-3 fatty acids. Sardines packed in sardine oil contain the most. The can will be labeled "Sild Sardine Oil." Sild sardines are young herring imported from Norway.

Are You a Seafood Lover?

Nutritionists say fish are nutrient-dense. They are rich in B vitamins as well as being good sources of phosphorus, potassium, and iron. Salt-water fish provide iodine and cancer-fighting selenium.

As we noted in a previous chapter, shellfish are one of the richest sources of zinc. Oysters, shrimp, clams, and unboned, canned fish such as sardines and salmon are also high in bone-building calcium. Eating fish may even prevent cavities since they supply significant amounts of fluoride to anyone living without fluoridated water.

Of course, for the dieter, seafoods are a great source of low-calorie protein. For example, a three and one-half ounce cooked portion of white fish provides about one-third of an adult's daily need for protein and is low in calories (less than 100).

Most seafoods are now known to be low in cholesterol. Even those that were thought to be cholesterol-carriers— shrimp, crab, and lobster—have now been cleared of any real harmfulness since they contain less cholesterol per serving than one egg.

What About Fish Pills?

If you read magazines, I am sure you've seen the recent ads promoting fish oil capsules. Fish oil may help lower blood pressure, relieve skin disorders such as eczema and psoriasis, combat some of the age-related protein deposits that cause organs to malfunction, help with arthritis, and aid brain development.

As a result of this new evidence, drug manufacturers are extracting fish oil as fast as they can and putting it on the market in capsules. Many of the companies doing this are reporting sensational sales not only in health food stores but in regular food stores as well.

The question is: Are they any good? The American Medical Association and the American Heart Association say, "No!" Both associations recommend including generous portions of fish in your diet, but they state that not enough is known about the fish oil capsule for it to be marketed yet.

Fish oil prevents clotting of the blood. This could make the fish oil capsules dangerous by hampering proper clotting of blood in case of accidents. Too much fish oil can lead to a deficiency of Vitamin E.

Experts are not sure whether the omega-3s, alone, are responsible for the nutritional benefits of fish. They say it could be a combination of several elements in the fish working with the omega-3s to bring about the benefits.

You will continue to see the fish oil capsules for sale. But if you want to wait and see what researchers say before you take them, you are wise. In the meantime, eat more fish.

Lengthen Your Life

Cholesterol ranks among the top three contributors to heart disease. Like high blood pressure and smoking, cholesterol can be controlled through modifications in diet. If heart disease runs in your family, get your cholesterol checked and under control.

Cut down on saturated fats by substituting fish and chicken for red meats, include foods that actually lower cholesterol in your diet, and exercise sensibly. You can make changes that will improve the quality and the length of your life.

——24——
Protecting Yourself Against Cancer

Every few months we hear another report, "Recent findings indicate bacon causes cancer." Fried hamburgers cause cancer. Red dye. Decaffeinated coffee. Regular coffee. Maybe we should ask what *doesn't* cause cancer rather than what does. The list of forbidden foods and substances seems to be endless. What can a person do? Quit living? Quit eating?

We undoubtedly live in a high-risk environment when it comes to cancer. But there are some very logical steps we can take to reduce the risks. Both the American Cancer Society and the National Cancer Institute are launching dietary programs of attack against cancer. Their aim is to save lives through nutritional education. The medical community has finally begun to support the idea that the right diet may help prevent cancer.

You can reduce the risk of cancer by staying slim, eating lots of fruits and vegetables, cutting fat from your diet, and abstaining from alcohol and cigarettes.

The Link Between Cancer and Fat

Excess weight, fat intake, and overeating seem to make a person cancer-prone. Researchers have found unusually high cancer rates among the obese. Studies seem to indicate that fats and oils promote cancer.

Americans consume more than sixty pounds of oil annually, and it is killing us. Few of us would add twelve teaspoons of butter to an eight-ounce baked potato, but that's what happens when potatoes become potato chips.

Almost 250,000 women this year can expect to be diagnosed as having one of the four major fatal cancers in women—breast, lung, uterine, or colorectal. Almost 100,000 will die from one of these.

Studies link breast cancer and fat. Breast cancer affects one out of every ten American women. Early detection is the key to survival once it occurs. More than 75 percent of all breast cancers are detected through self-examination.

The best advice for those who want to avoid breast cancer is to follow a low-fat diet and have a mammogram at least every two years between the ages of thirty-five and forty-nine and every year after age fifty.

Links between certain hormones and fat increase the risk of breast cancer. Scientists don't fully understand why, but fat seems to affect the hormone balance of the body by triggering an increase in the production of estrogen.

Roughly 75 percent of all breast cancers occur in post-menopausal women over age fifty whose main source of estrogen is fat tissue in the breast, hips, and thighs. The older and more overweight a woman is, the more estrogen her fat tissue forms.

The National Cancer Institute blames fatty foods for breast cancer. White fat itself does not cause cancer but seems to promote the development of tumors caused by other substances. Researchers suspect this because the cancers form only when fat, among other factors, is present.

Cancer-Preventative Diet

The American Cancer Society states that diet plays a part in 35 percent of all cancer cases in the United States.

Evidence suggests that changed eating habits can certainly reduce occurrence of colon and breast cancer, which now kills some 50,000 and 40,000 Americans respectively each year. Lung cancer kills some 120,000 each year.

A low-fat diet means low-risk to your health. Here are dietary recommendations from the American Cancer Society.

1. Eat less fat. Adjust your calorie intake to maintain an ideal body weight. Allow no more than 30 percent of your calories to be fat. Low-fat ways to prepare food include steaming, poaching, stir-frying, broiling, baking, microwaving, and grilling.

2. Eat more high-fiber food such as fruits, vegetables, and whole-grain cereal.

3. Eat foods rich in vitamins A and C.

4. Eat "cruciferous" vegetables such as cabbage, broccoli, brussels sprouts, and cauliflower.

5. If you drink alcohol, do so in moderation. No more than two drinks a day.

6. Eat less salt-cured, smoked, and nitrite-treated food.

7. Eat less altogether and avoid being overweight.

Foods that Protect Against Cancer

Oatmeal is a good disease-fighting breakfast food that wards off heart disease by lowering blood pressure and cholesterol levels in the blood. The water-soluble fibers in oats help stabilize blood sugar levels in diabetics. Some experts think a high-fiber diet may even be a factor in preventing diabetes.

Oat bran and other fibers are natural digestive-tract aids that will keep your weight down by providing stomach-satisfying bulk at a low-calorie cost. A three-fourths cup serving of quick-cooked oatmeal made only with water has 108 calories.

Broccoli and other members of the "cabbage family" protect against cancer because they contain substances that block the formation of cancer-causing chemicals in the body. People who frequently eat these vegetables are much less likely to develop cancers of the digestive tract. A large stalk of cooked broccoli has only 26 calories. Broccoli is also a rich source of vitamin A, which helps protects against cancer.

By eating just three carrots a week, you can meet your body's need for vitamin A and protect yourself from cancer in the process. Carrots contain beta-carotene, a substance used by the body to manufacture vitamin A. There is strong evidence that beta-carotene helps prevent the development of cancers in certain tissues throughout the body such as the lungs, breasts, and digestive tract.

Recent research indicates that red foods—tomatoes, strawberries, cranberries, watermelon, and pink grapefruit—all contain lycopene, a red pigment that may help protect against cancer. Lycopene is part of the carotenoid family of substances that seem to offer cancer protection. The best known, as we mentioned above, is beta-carotene.

Somehow lycopene acts as a detoxifier of the oxygen-free radicals that have been thought to cause cancer. Although scientist still are not sure just what it is in green and red vegetables and fruits that protect against cancer, it's a safe bet that you will benefit from eating them.

Fiber and Cancer Prevention

Studies reveal that people who eat more fiber are less likely to get colon cancer. Fiber empties the colon faster and removes carcinogens before the body can absorb them. Excess fats in the diet also stimulate production of bile acids. Bile acids and fatty acids are connected to colon cancer. Bran fiber dilutes these bile and fatty acids as does calcium in milk.

Studies by the National Cancer Institute of populations with low incidence of colon cancer have revealed fiber to be the reason. People in Finland, for example, eat a high-fat, high-fiber diet and have a low incidence of colon cancer.

Other groups who eat high-fiber diets are Mormons, Seventh-Day Adventists, and the third world countries. They don't all eat the same kind of fiber—some eat fresh fruits and vegetables, others consume wheat-grain-type fibers.

The ratio of fiber to fat probably makes the difference between a high and low incidence of colon cancer. All experts in the field believe that adding fiber to your diet will reduce not only the risk of colon cancer but breast and lung cancer as well.

Fighting cancer doesn't have to be hard. There are some simple changes you can make to protect yourself.

1. Avoid cigarettes, caffeine, alcohol, and artificial sweeteners completely.

2. Eat salted and pickled foods, browned foods, fat, and protein in strictest moderation.

3. Avoid charring foods in the browning process. This creates substances called mutagens that have produced cancer in laboratory animals.

4. Eat plenty of fresh fruits and vegetables, especially oranges, apples, carrots, broccoli, cabbage, and cauliflower—all fibrous food.

Cancer and Calcium

One study by two California scientists shows a possible connection between calcium deficiency and cancer.

In looking at maps showing where the different types of cancer were most prevalent throughout the country, the scientists noticed that there was a definite geographical pattern to the maps showing incidence of breast cancer and intestinal cancer. The area north of the fortieth parallel or that area north of Arizona, New Mexico, Texas, Tennessee, and the Carolinas showed the highest breast and intestinal cancer mortality rates. The Sunbelt areas showed a low-cancer rate for breast and intestinal cancer.

They determined that no geographical differences in food consumption could account for this. Researchers discovered the death rate from breast cancer was higher in cities than in rural areas. Evidence pointed to sunlight as the key factor.

Sunlight reacts with cholesterol inside and on the surface of the skin to create vitamin D. Vitamin D, as learned earlier, helps the body absorb calcium.

Once vitamin D reaches the small intestine, it directs the cells lining the intestine to produce a calcium-binding protein that lies in wait and hooks any calcium passing by. This calcium is carried everywhere it is needed in the body including the breasts and intestine. Without vitamin D much calcium is wasted or eliminated.

Calcium carries messages between the cells of body tissue. If calcium is too low, the cells fail to communicate correctly, the tissue becomes disorganized, and the stage is set for cancer. Other studies have also revealed evidence that calcium is essential to cancer prevention.

Walk Away from Cancer

Can physical fitness help prevent cancer? Studies of women who competed in basketball, swimming, tennis, track, gymnastics, and other sports in college showed that women who maintained their activity level developed half the cancer of the breast and female organs as their sedentary counterparts.

Other studies have shown that men with physically-active jobs were less likely to develop colon cancer than those with office-type jobs. Because of the evidence that physical activity reduces cancer, the American Cancer Society now recommends exercise as a preventive measure.

In animal studies, rats were given a chemical that causes breast cancer. Half the rats were put in cages with free access to an exercise wheel, allowing them to run anytime they wished. The other group was not allowed to exercise.

The rats with access to the wheel developed one-third fewer cases of cancer than the inactive rats. The tumors that the active rats developed appeared much later than the lesions in their sedentary counterparts.

How does exercise fight cancer? Primarily, exercise fights body fat, forces the body to dip into its energy reserves, and converts stored protein into usable glucose. Some researchers think that hormones used to initiate this process provide the body with cancer protection. Studies also reveal that exercise stimulates the body's cancer-fighting immune system. More studies have to be done, but enough evidence exists to encourage anyone to exercise.

Is Cancer Hereditary?

Only five to seven percent of all cancer is hereditary in nature. Most cancer stems from environmental factors such as diet, smoking, chemical exposure, and radiation.

If your close relatives have had cancer, however, your risk is much higher. For example, if both your mother and sister have had breast cancer, then you have fourteen times the normal risk of developing the same.

This would also apply to colon cancer. Colon cancer is not inherited, but polyps are. If polyps are in your family history, have your physician check your colon for any incidence of them. If they occur, have them removed in order to avoid the risk of cancer.

You cannot do much about your height, your eye color, or your skin color, but you can do something about your health. You do not have to follow the same health patterns as your relatives, particularly if those patterns were bad. Through moderation in lifestyle, diet, and exercise, you can direct the course of your health to a great extent. Chronic diseases take a long time to develop, which means you have time to do something about them. With proper action you can help avoid a disease that has run in your family for many generations.

─────25─────
PMS, Pregnancy, and Menopause

I recently received a phone call from a very frustrated young woman. Like myself, she had a public ministry. Her ministry involved singing for the Lord on a television program and through personal appearances in churches.

Her phone call was motivated by a terrible depression that had carried over into her marriage and ministry. A complete physical examination revealed nothing unusual, but her doctor surmised the depression was probably caused by a hormonal imbalance in her system.

I asked Ann a few questions to discover if she was taking birth control pills or some other medication that would affect the hormonal system of her body. Next, I asked how she felt about herself. That question opened a deluge of troubles and frustrations. Carrying 130 pounds on her five foot frame, Ann absolutely hated her appearance. Desperate to lose her excess baggage, Ann had tried not to eat at all but found herself starving and binging.

"I go wild and eat five or six candy bars at a time," she lamented. "I feel like an animal. Once I start eating, I can't stop. If there's anything in the house, I have to eat it. Once I stop eating, I hate myself and just want to cry."

Before her monthly cycle Ann craved all kinds of sweet and salty foods. She also would go to pieces, yell at her husband, and shake. Had her doctor suggested an exercise program? No, he had not. I told her a daily commitment to exercise was exactly what she needed for her mental and physical condition. I believe her symptoms were, to a great degree, caused by a lack of exercise.

My Advice

I advised her to devote one and one-half hours a day to exercise. Ann agreed to walk briskly first thing every morning. Following her walk, she would work out with me during my program. As soon as she could do the exercises, I suggested she add a one-pound weight to each wrist and each ankle to speed muscle development. In the evenings, Ann would either take another thirty-minute walk or use her exercise bike for thirty minutes.

Why so much exercise? First, Ann needs to lose weight. The one-hour walking program will burn fat. The thirty-minute floor workout with me will improve her posture, flexibility, and muscle mass, as well as strengthen her lower back and flatten her stomach. During my program I will share nutrition information with Ann and encourage her to exercise. So often this is exactly what a person needs to stay motivated.

In my daily television show, I constantly teach my audience about all the wonderful changes going on in their bodies that scales can't measure—like the reduction in fat, the increase in muscle mass, and heightened metabolism. Scales just measure up and down. They cannot tell you if your loss is fat or fluid.

In Ann's case, she was trying to reduce by starving herself. Her body rebelled and caused the uncontrollable binging. As a result, depression and low self-esteem plagued this fine Christian woman and hindered her testimony.

I encouraged Ann to go on a low-fat diet of fruits, vegetables, and whole grains. These complex carbohydrates made up 55 percent of her diet, fat was no more than 30 percent, and protein comprised the balance.

On this regimen, Ann lost fifteen pounds, dropped three dress sizes, cured her binge eating, and conquered her depression. The exercise made her feel so much better. She gradually found it easier to eat right. "I don't want to expend all that energy and ruin it all by eating junk," she explained. Ann also avoided all sweet and salty foods and drank eight glasses of water each day.

In the end, her pre-menstrual symptoms were alleviated. The longer she stayed away from the sweets, the easier it became for her to avoid them. She learned that the body really prefers fresh fruit for dessert.

PMS: Fact or Fiction?

Ask any woman who has suffered with it, and she will tell you pre-menstrual syndrome (PMS) is real. This mysterious malady affects 90 percent of all women who are still menstruating and incapacitates a small percentage of them. Forty percent will tell you that PMS causes serious problems in their bodies and in their lives.

If you have two good weeks out of the month followed by two weeks of depression, irritability, headaches, swelling, bloating, anxiety, and food cravings, you are probably a PMS sufferer.

Here is one woman's typical reaction to her monthly symptoms. "I feel out of control. During the first two weeks of the month I follow a sound diet. But by the third week, I am craving sweet desserts and salty snacks. The week before my period I could eat chocolate all day. But once my period comes, the cravings disappear and I'm back to normal."

For a disease that carries 150 symptoms, little is actually known about PMS. I'm sure women have ended up in divorce court because of not knowing what to do about their PMS. How many others have been sent to a psychiatrist, put on tranquilizers, and misdiagnosed as being mentally ill when they were actually suffering a hormonal imbalance? PMS symptoms are easily mistaken for other problems.

I know one woman whose gynecologist sent her to a neurosurgeon rather than admit her headaches might be purely PMS-related and that he did not know how to help her. Even though this woman had headaches only during the two weeks prior to her period, he could not seem to accept PMS as a condition involving strictly the female system.

With no guidelines, little research, seemingly minimal interest by the medical profession as a whole, and not even any concrete proof that such a disease exists, doctors tend to underrate PMS or even ignore it. Physicians often blame the PMS symptoms on nerves or more-understood diseases. But women know PMS is a reality and a problem that can ruin their lives if it goes untreated.

Explaining PMS Symptoms

There are many theories as to what triggers the PMS response in women each month. Some say it is caused by having too much estrogen. Others say it's from having too little progesterone. Vitamin B deficiency, fluid retention, allergies, and mental illness also get the blame.

Although food cravings are not the only major PMS symptom, they are nevertheless part of the problem and can lead to weight gain. The reason for the food cravings is that a woman's appetite and her sex hormones share a common bond. One study showed that women ate 25 percent more for lunch just before menstruation.

Both estrogen and progesterone seem to influence your appetite and the regulation and distribution of fat cells. Estrogen seems to decrease hunger and progesterone seems to stimulate the appetite. Estrogen causes fat cells to store less fat and release it by metabolism.

After ovulation, the level of estrogen falls and the level of progesterone rises. Experts feel the monthly rise and fall of hormones are responsible for the many symptoms of PMS and also for the cravings experienced by pregnant women.

Stress and PMS

Perhaps the most frustrating words a PMS sufferer can hear is, "You must find a way to avoid stress." PMS is stress. Who can avoid stress anyway?

Since PMS occurs regularly during the two weeks prior to menstruation, a woman can know when to minimize stress in her life. A PMS sufferer can warn her husband, family, and friends what is happening in her body. When mood swings, depression, anger, and headaches occur, her support system can extend the extra patience, acceptance, and love that she needs. Family and friends can cope better by knowing the cause of a woman's tears, irritability, or strange behavior.

We can always resort to prayer for patience and the emotional stability found in Christ. God understands, and He wants to help. During those two weeks you may also want to increase your praise and worship time. No one can simultaneously worship and be focused on self. Search the Scriptures for words of comfort, strength, and peace during those trying times.

Progesterone seems to help some women some of the time. Birth control pills alleviate many of the symptoms for those women who don't mind the side effects of the pill such as sore breasts or nausea. Dietary changes and regular exercise can also help relieve stress and other PMS symptoms.

How To Handle PMS

So what can you do about PMS? First, don't feel guilty, abnormal, or think that you're crazy. Although no one understands the cause of those symptoms, realize that you're suffering a hormonal imbalance. You did not make it up. Second, diet control and exercise can go a long way in minimizing the symptoms.

Here are some doctor-recommended tips on handling PMS:

1. Try eating six small meals each day rather than three large ones.
2. Follow a low-fat, high complex-carbohydrate diet rich in whole-grain breads, cereals, fresh vegetables, and beans.
3. Reduce intake of red meat by substituting low-fat chicken and fish.
4. Reduce salt intake.
5. Avoid sweets.
6. Reduce or eliminate caffeine and alcohol intake.
7. Exercise an hour each day.

Since exercise stimulates beta-endorphins (the euphoric-type chemical produced in the brain during exercise), it will relieve some of the anxiety and depression associated with PMS. Vigorous exercise such as walking briskly will work wonders for the PMS sufferer.

New drugs are on the market, but the best "cure" for PMS is proper diet and exercise. Remember that water is the best diuretic for combatting fluid retention no matter what its cause. Drinking six to eight glasses of water each day is absolutely essential for the PMS sufferer.

Pregnancy and Weight Gain

During pregnancy more than any other time in her life, a woman must carefully plan for her health and diet. Through good nutrition, a mother can give her baby a first-rate start in life. Eating for two is perfectly healthy during pregnancy. A mother-to-be must consume enough calories so her baby will be large enough at birth to survive.

Years ago doctors stressed keeping weight down during pregnancy. Believe it or not, this idea originated in the nineteenth century when an epidemic of rickets caused a narrowing of hips in women. Doctors severely limited weight gain during pregnancy so the babies could move through the pelvis of the mothers.

Somehow this idea carried over into the 1960s and 1970s. But now, thank goodness, doctors are insisting that mothers eat and eat for two. Skipping meals during pregnancy can cause the body to produce certain harmful chemicals that could lead to fetal brain disorders.

Don't be upset if you gain more than the average of 25 or 30 pounds. Don't "pig out" the whole nine months, but do eat well-balanced meals. Doctors are now saying it is better to gain more weight than not enough. You wouldn't miss a feeding after the baby is born, would you? So you shouldn't miss a feeding before the baby is born, either.

What if you're already carrying excess poundage when you discover you're pregnant? Even an overweight woman should plan to gain during pregnancy. No one should lose weight during those very important nine months. If you do, something is wrong.

Needed Nutrients During Pregnancy

In our weight-conscious society, getting expectant mothers to eat right has become a real problem. The baby grows on what the mother eats, not on what she stores as fat. The body is all set to help the mother and baby survive if the mother will cooperate. If a mother doesn't eat enough, deformities and problems can result in her malnourished baby.

Some of the nutrients crucial to a healthy pregnancy are iron, calcium, zinc, and folic acid. A pregnant woman needs more iron because her blood volume is increasing.

Sufficient calcium intake is vital during pregnancy. If the baby can't absorb calcium through the normal routes, it will deplete the mother's own calcium reserve, causing osteoporosis later in life.

A woman's body absorbs calcium twice as well during pregnancy. Since estrogen levels are high during pregnancy, if you have plenty of calcium in your diet, you can actually build bone tissue during this time.

Folic acid is found in liver and green leafy vegetables. Your doctor will tell you if you need a multi-vitamin supplement and what kind to get. Most physicians recommend this.

Preventing Birth Defects

If you are pregnant or thinking of becoming pregnant, protect your unborn child in every way possible. Amazingly, educated and intelligent women are still confused as to what they should or should not be eating, drinking, and breathing during pregnancy.

A slight risk of some sort of genetic disorder exists with any pregnancy. But even when the risk is present—and sometimes against all odds—most babies are born healthy. The chances are good that you will have a normal baby. What can you do to prevent any unnecessary risks? Here are some tips for the expectant mother.

Don't drink alcohol at all while pregnant or even if you suspect you are. You don't have to be an alcoholic to give birth to a child that has been severely damaged by alcohol. A university study has shown that pregnant women who had as few as two drinks a week could give birth to infants with such problems as high tension, stomach upset, and withdrawal symptoms. Withdrawal symptoms occur with alcohol as well as drugs.

You don't have to be an alcoholic to give birth to a baby with fetal alcohol syndrome (FAS). Characteristics of a baby born with FAS include abnormally small head, deformed facial features, mental retardation, poor coordination, and sometimes heart defects. FAS, present in one out of every

750 babies born today, is the third most common cause of mental retardation in the United States. Unlike genetic disorders beyond the control of parents, FAS can be prevented.

Since no one knows how much alcohol is too much during pregnancy, the best thing you can do for your child and yourself is to totally avoid it. If you cannot give up alcohol, don't get pregnant.

Having a Healthy Baby

Studies show that cigarette smokers give birth to smaller babies who are prone to infection and diseases. Nearly one-half of all newborn deaths occur with low-weight infants.

Smoking is also known to cause miscarriage, stillbirth, and premature birth. At least one study has shown that the children of smokers have more learning difficulties. Smoking actually causes the blood vessels leading to the baby to constrict. If the mother smokes enough, blood flow to the fetus can be compromised.

Do yourself and your baby a favor. Quit smoking and never take it back up again. Smoking can be especially harmful during the last week before delivery when babies need all the oxygen the mother can provide.

Never take any drugs of any kind without your doctor's knowledge and consent during pregnancy. If you can possibly get along without all medicines during this time, do. Even though your doctor will let you take Tylenol if needed, any other medication is better left alone.

Staying Fit During Pregnancy

Staying fit during pregnancy has limitless physical and psychological benefits. You can pretty much follow your normal exercise routine once you have cleared it with your doctor. Just avoid bouncing or rapid, jerky movements.

Expectant mothers must also know when to stop. In an aerobic workout, fifteen minutes is enough.

During pregnancy it is more important than ever to drink water before, during, and after exercise. Overheating can trigger premature labor.

Will exercise give you an easier delivery? There is no evidence that it will, but you will be in better mental and physical shape. I personally believe that exercise will make the delivery easier and the labor even shorter because I feel it did for me.

Consult your doctor about all exercise routines as soon as you know you are pregnant. Don't begin any new exercise program once you discover you're expecting. Avoid all exercises for the abdominal area during pregnancy as well.

Dealing with Menopause

On my forty-sixth birthday, I had my last menstrual period. Had I known that was my last one, I might have felt very sad. You see, I picture myself as a child. I'm so grateful to God that I can roll myself into a little ball, jump right up, and run for miles and miles. With all my strength and energy, I just can't help but feel young. When it finally dawned on me that I was experiencing change of life, I started to think, "I'm getting old."

When I visited my doctor a few months later, he told me that very fit women commonly enter menopause early. What symptoms had I noticed? I had experienced nothing other than a brief "hot spell" that soon passed.

I decided that this was just another stage in my life, and I wanted to approach it with an open mind. I even thought, "Now I'll be able to share even more things with my viewers." I haven't experienced any real discomfort. Not having a period for a while seemed strange, but now I've grown used to it.

I'm very much aware of my need to drink skim milk and take a calcium supplement. Because I didn't drink milk during my twenties and early thirties, I know that calcium loss could be a real problem for me.

Following a good, healthy diet and regular, daily exercise is absolutely essential to my good health. When I was younger, I could cheat on weekends and enjoy fattening desserts. But realizing that my health is my responsibility, I must eat smart at all times to nourish my body. If you adapt this same lifestyle, you'll also reap the benefits of health, energy, and vitality.

When Was Your Last Check-Up?

Annual physicals are necessary for preventing and detecting health problems. As we get older, we need to have our cholesterol, blood pressure, and other aspects of our health checked on a regular basis.

For a number of years I did not have a check-up, but now that I am forty-six, I really believe in annual physicals. Last year my doctor discovered several masses in my breast tissue, so I had two mammograms performed. A tumor can easily hide behind a mass of tissue, so early detection is one of the best ways to beat breast cancer. Monthly self-examination can prevent you from being a statistic.

Since there is a history of colon cancer in my family, my doctor put me through a series of tests for that, too. You may think tests are inconvenient, but remember that early detection can save your life.

Maintaining proper weight helps you be aware of your body, which enables you to quickly detect when something is wrong. I have friends who have detected the very early stages of cancer because they were so "in tune" with their bodies through exercise.

Excess weight can cover up a fatal disease. You can feel so badly that you don't even realize your condition is worsening. Even surgery is more difficult when individuals are overweight. For your health's sake, stay on a low-fat diet coupled with regular exercise.

Minimizing the Symptoms

Many times with the onset of menopause, a woman will notice that her skin becomes drier and her hair begins to thin. These changes are nothing to be worried about. A few tips can help you minimize the effect of these symptoms.

Using a moisture-rich soap rather than a harsh deodorant soap is so important. Deodorant soaps will dry out the skin. Soaking in a hot tub of water will dehydrate skin as well. When you bathe, use warm water (not hot) and a moisture-rich bath oil. After bathing, use lotion on the body and a rich moisturizer on the face and neck. This will prevent water loss through the skin and keep skin soft.

Above all, during outdoor activities of any measurable length, use a sunscreen. The sun damages the skin far more than menopause.

Some menopausal women experience severe dryness of hands that leads to deep cracks in the skin. If moisturizers do not help, see your doctor about using a steroid cream.

Hair should receive gentle treatment at all times. Using a conditioner slows down damage by preventing breakage. Perms should be avoided if possible. Space them out to give your hair a break from the strong chemical solutions. Hot curlers and combs should be used sparingly. Anything that pulls or heats your scalp can lead to hair loss.

There is also a drug called minoxidil, which helps slow hair loss, but must be used under the care of a doctor. If you have noticed a hair loss, check with your doctor because hair loss can also be a sign of thyroid problems.

Menopause triggers a loss of hormones, especially estrogen, and can affect a woman's looks. Hot flashes can ruin the complexion and ruin restful sleep. Lack of good sleep deepens wrinkles and increases signs of aging.

Estrogen Replacement Therapy can bring back balance and help a woman regain her energy and natural good looks. ERT helps reverse the loss of collagen, which gives elasticity to the skin. Not every woman can have ERT, and those who do must be regularly checked by their doctors.

With a good attitude and some practical advice, most women can tackle the challenges of PMS, pregnancy, and menopause. A sound diet and daily exercise makes sense for a woman at every stage of her life.

Part Five
On Your Way

—————26—————
Aging Gracefully

A woman told her doctor that with each birthday, she became more and more terrified at the thought of growing old. "I feel my self-image dwindling with each passing year," she lamented. "As people around me seem to look younger and younger, I feel that I look older and older."

Perhaps our society places too high a value on youth and not enough on life after forty. Prevailing attitudes contribute to the uneasiness women feel about the aging process. Society and the media have made a natural, beautiful transition look like a terrible disease or something to be shunned.

Those over forty are led to believe that they are dull, uninteresting, and have lost their appeal. This is far from true. I believe we're only learning how to make the most of life at forty. In many ways life does begin at forty, especially for the person who has learned to live healthy, live for others, and exercise the mind and body.

Staying Young at Heart

Our society may be moving away from its preoccupation with youth and is beginning to accord dignity, respect, and happiness to aging. Thank God for the signs of change on the horizon! We must see beauty in life and humanity at all stages of our lives.

I believe that life can be even better after forty than it was before. Your children are usually close to being grown. You have more time to pursue your own interests and to take care of yourself.

We need to fill our lives with new and good experiences. New experiences destroy the illusion that life is passing us by. If you feel life has nothing new to offer, search for some fresh undertaking or venture. Sure, risks may be involved, but risks are exciting. Yes, there will be some anxiety at the changes you will go through, but as you begin to live again, the anxiety will diminish with each new challenge.

Success more often than not is a process of trial and error. Have you always wanted your own craft shop or your own business? Have you always wanted to reach out and help those in nursing homes or hospitals? Expand your world. Open your own business. Be a volunteer at the nursing home or hospital. Go back to school. Travel. Try a new hobby. Eat healthy and exercise.

Through change we grow and learn. Learning is another way to offset aging and keep excitement and vitality. Be in control of the aging process instead of letting it control you.

Minimizing the Aging Process

Women are especially affected by what they see in their own mirror. Our appearance counts at any age. Beginning in middle age when wrinkles and sags begin to change your familiar face into one you don't know, depression all too frequently follows.

The physical evidence of aging can be offset through exercise, diet, clever make-up, hairstyle, and color. Some women can accept gray hair and lines with ease and grace. Others are devastated by them and need ways to minimize them. Knowing and understanding yourself and your needs can help you cope with aging.

Two new terms regarding aging have cropped up recently. They are primary aging and secondary aging. *Primary aging* is a natural fact of life. *Secondary aging* is aging that occurs, not as a result of years, but as a result of inactivity.

As people grow older they often become less active. Somehow the myth that aging means slowing down has never been eradicated. This very "slowing down" actually accelerates the aging process. Much aging is really a result of inactivity and poor diet. Someone has rightly said that more people die of disuse than old age. Don't ever think you are too old or too fat to exercise.

With good health practices, lots of exercise, and a positive outlook on life, you can actually look younger. Faith in God shows on your countenance and takes years off your face. Taking those cares to the Lord in prayer and communing with Him can give you a merrier heart and a happier face. God magnificently created our bodies to respond if we start taking care of them. Just thank God for what you are able to do today and think positively about yourself.

Can Diet Slow Aging?

We need certain amounts of nutrients each day in order to live our normal life spans. If a certain combination of foods keeps us healthy, would it not stand to reason that a better combination might keep us healthy even longer?

Experts now believe that manipulating the diet can actually slow the aging process, especially in such areas as bone thinning, hardening of the arteries, and a declining immune system. Certain nutrients produce a drug-like effect that may prevent some of the most life-threatening diseases.

The more attention we pay to good nutrition, the more we slow the aging process. As we grow older our metabolic rate slows, and we need less fuel to support our activities. People age fifty-five and older, for example, need 150 to 200 less calories per day than people between the ages of thirty-five and fifty-five.

While our bodies need less food as we grow older, we need more highly nutritious food. In other words, the food you eat must carry a lot of nutritional power. Every calorie must be nutritious as age advances past fifty-five.

Because kidney function is reduced with age, eating less protein will ease stress on your kidneys and your pocketbook. Protein is expensive, and we need far less than we eat.

While you need less protein after age fifty-five, you need more dietary fiber, iron, and vitamin B-12. The need for calcium was covered in an earlier chapter, and it is vital to your good health at any age.

Fish Oil and Aging

In an earlier chapter we talked about cold-water fish and their omega-3 fat that helps lower cholesterol levels in the bloodstream. New research is indicating that this same fish oil helps combat or slow the aging process.

One of the agents that ages the body is a protein called amyloid, which is deposited in the heart, kidneys, and other organs and is also connected to arthritis. Fish oil apparently slows the build-up of amyloids in the body. This is just one more reason to include salmon, mackerel, and other cold-water fish in your regular diet.

Sunlight and Your Body

The skin is the body's vitamin D factory, and the factory must have sunlight in order to work right. As skin ages, it becomes less and less able to provide the body with vitamin D. The older person needs twice as much sun to meet the body's vitamin D needs as a teenager does.

The aging process also hampers the body's ability to digest milk and milk products. Milk gradually becomes less a source of vitamin D. Bone damage is the inevitable result.

To insure you get enough vitamin D, try to be in direct sunlight at least twenty minutes each day and include egg yolks, liver, and tuna in your diet. Consult your doctor about a vitamin D supplement.

Muscle Mass, Metabolism, and Aging

So many people ask, "Why do I tend to put on weight as I get older even though I am eating as I always have?"

The standard answer is that metabolism slows down with age. Studies have shown that as it grows older, the human body continues to burn calories at the same rate per pound of muscle. The key phrase is "per pound of muscle." That's where the catch is. Muscle tissue burns calories when a person is active and at rest.

As we age, we tend to be less active and thus lose much of our muscle mass. With less muscle available to burn calories, fewer of the calories we eat get burned up. Those not burned are stored in the body as fat, and fat doesn't burn calories at all.

Would weight lifting exercises benefit the person over forty? Muscle growth for the older individual will not be as significant as it is for the younger exerciser. Older individuals can expect some increase in muscle size from weight training, but a younger person would experience more.

The good news is that an older weight lifter can achieve almost as much increase in strength as he could when he was younger. Why? As we grow older, we are better at learning to activate the nerves that make muscle fibers contract.

A comparison of strength of one hundred men doing similar work in a machine shop showed no significant difference between the strength of twenty-two-year-olds and sixty-two-year-olds. Loss in strength with age is attributed primarily to disuse rather than any effect of aging.

How to Combat Aging

According to the medical opinion of the American Geriatrics Association, problems frequently diagnosed as aging are actually muscle disease. Exercise should be the standard remedy for aging and should be prescribed as such by doctors.

How much of aging is aging and how much is attributed to abuses of the body?

I believe the decline in kidney function, bone density, flexibility, circulation, and lung capacity is more a result of inactivity and improper dietary practices than it is aging. Excesses of alcohol, smoking, and stress can also contribute to premature aging.

I know women in their fifties and sixties who have begun to take years off their bodies and faces through exercise and diet. The combination of mental and physical well-being brings about a younger appearance. Inactivity seems to be the culprit in aging. You can be twenty years old but look and feel like you are forty.

Here are some ways exercise combats aging:

1. Improves flexibility and mobility.
2. Improves breathing.
3. Strengthens the heart and lungs.
4. Decreases blood pressure, body fat, and bone loss.
5. Improves self-esteem and appearance.

The older we are, the harder we must work at firming and toning muscles. But studies have shown that even moderate exercise can prolong life. Inactive lifestyles lead to heart and lung diseases. Large numbers of Americans are dying simply from inactivity.

Are We Really Helping?

Many times we think we're helping our parents or grand-parents by saying, "Don't get up, Mother. I'll do that for you." If we really did what was best for her, we would say, "Yes, get up, Mother. Move around. Do all you possibly can to keep going."

If someone you love is a senior citizen, or if you are, encourage them to mow the grass, rake the yard, or even vacuum if they want to. Let them plant and tend a garden. Quit cringing and trying to shield them from any physical exertion. Realize that exercise is necessary for good health. People who sit down at age sixty-five and reduce their lifestyle to strolls to the bathroom, bed, porch, or kitchen are also taking a short stroll to an early grave.

The elderly should not be expected to work like a young person or do more than their doctors permit. But they must do all they possibly can to remain active. Activity will allow them independence and dignity, and they will feel good about themselves. Everyone needs to feel worthwhile, useful, and needed. Show your love by letting your elderly friends and family be active and useful.

Certain studies have indicated that both the physical and mental condition of the elderly improves with exercise. Forty-eight seniors with an average age of seventy-two were tested and assigned to an exercise group or a non-exercise group. The exercisers showed improved heart rate, weight loss, and increased flexibility. They also reported feelings of personal mastery, of having more control over their lives, and a decrease in depression and anxiety. Improvements in problem-solving, memory, and concentration were reported.

Good Posture and Aging

Good posture will slow the aging process and improve your health. Yet posture remains off the list of many exercise programs. At least one doctor believes that good posture can even reverse the aging process.

Few of us have time to walk around with a book on our head. Many of us try to remember the time-honored rules of good posture: tuck in buttocks, square shoulders, and hold in the tummy. These exercises, however, are too hard to maintain over long periods of time.

Experts say the most natural way to control posture is with your head. Your head weighs ten to fifteen pounds. When it slumps forward, the rest of you is out of kilter. If your head slumps forward, you lose the ability to move your neck properly, which can eventually lead to arthritis in the neck joints.

Bad posture also results in fatigue, bursitis, depleted lung capacity, gastrointestinal problems, and TMJ (a painful jaw problem). Poor posture usually reveals a poor self-image.

Improving your posture is a simple matter. Stand with your back to a wall, knees bent, and feet flat on the floor. Place your hands beside your head with your elbows touching the wall. Don't raise your hands suddenly or forcefully.

Tilt your pelvis and flatten your lower back against the wall by tucking in your tummy area. Do this for five or ten seconds each day and soon you'll be in "good standing." Of course, you can always use the book-on-the-head method. Instead of the book, a bean bag does the same job and will stay on your head better.

Correct posture and exercise usually go hand in hand. Red blood cells are formed in the bone marrow and any skeletal imbalances in your body can restrict blood flow and hinder bone function.

As we grow older, we lose height because our necks tend to curve forward and the upper back becomes rounded. This tendency can be slowed and even stopped with exercise. Research has shown that if physical activity is slowed, the long bones stop making red blood cells. Bones respond and function better with activity.

The Skin and Aging

A woman wrote to a beauty consultant and extolled the wonderful effect exercise had on her body as far as slowing the aging process. Her skin, however, was continuing to age at a much faster rate than the rest of her. For many women, the skin is the first to go. What can be done to slow this process?

Perhaps the most common type of wrinkles are from expression lines such as the lines between the brow. These are caused by overuse of the facial muscles. Where the constant use of other muscles in your body will tone and firm them, the use of facial muscles just causes a lining of the face. This is because facial muscles attach to the skin. Other muscles attach to bone.

Frowning and smiling pulls at the skin and eventually leads to frown and laugh lines. Facial tension occurs quite easily. Just concentrating on reading material can bring an unconscious frown to your face. Learn to consciously relax your facial muscles. This will help prevent new lines from forming but will not eradicate those already present. Only cosmetic surgery can do that.

Exercising and Your Skin

Can exercise slow aging of the skin? Experts tell us that exercisers have healthier skin than non-exercisers. In a Finnish study, middle-aged athletes were found to have thicker, more dense, more elastic, less-wrinkled skin than counterparts who were sedentary. The increased blood flow to the skin during exercise may account for these factors.

Exercise also raises the temperature of the skin, which increases the amount of collagen produced. Collagen is the skin's support structure or elasticity, and exercise keeps collagen thick and strong. If we do not exercise, the support structure grows thin and weak with age.

Keeping the skin clean on the outside is not enough. Through vigorous exercise, skin can be cleansed from the inside out. Exercise opens up the capillaries that run directly under the skin, increases the amount of blood flowing through the skin, and carries more oxygen and nutrients to the skin and more waste material away from it.

Tips on Skin Care

Your skin is the largest organ of your body. It must be kept clean and protected. Nothing beats soap and water for cleansing the skin. Water should be warm or cool but not hot. Soaps should be mild.

Here's a list of suggestions on how to help your skin and protect it from premature aging:

1. Use a good moisturizer. After a shower or bath, apply moisturizer within three minutes. After that time, any water added to the skin will begin to evaporate and take some of your skin's own moisture with it. Your skin will end up being drier than when you started unless you apply moisturizer while the skin is still damp.

2. Drink at least three 12-ounce glasses of water a day. This is the absolute bare minimum for moist skin.

3. Don't overdo it in the sun. Today's gorgeous tan will line your face one day with a web of wrinkles. When in the sun, use sunscreens to protect against aging and skin cancer. Twenty minutes of direct sunlight a day is plenty for your vitamin D needs.

4. Exercise daily for at least thirty to forty-five minutes.

5. Keep your skin clean.

6. Keep cosmetics to a minimum. Wear the least amount you can to look your best.

7. Sleep on your back. Pillows and the mattress can crease your face and tug at your skin.

8. Learn to consciously relax facial muscles.

The Thymus Gland and Aging

Many years ago, scientists discovered that as people grew older, their organ weights changed. The lungs, liver, and brain weighed slightly less in an eighty-year-old than in a twenty-year-old. The thymus gland, however, shrinks to a tiny portion of its original size as age advances.

What is the thymus gland? This flat, pinkish-gray, two-lobed gland lies high in the chest behind the lungs and breast bone. They also found that the thymus gland distributes white blood cells and nourishes them with its hormones.

White blood cells, if you recall, fight disease. The white blood cells get their orders from the thymus gland. The thymus also seems to activate and command macrophages, cells that aid in the fight against disease.

But as the thymus shrinks with age, the body has less help in its fight against disease. Certain scientists believe that is why illness, cancer, infection, and death increase with age.

Research has also shown that diet can have a tremendous effect on the shrinking of the thymus, therefore affecting the aging of the body's immune system. Since the thymus is full of zinc, it stands to reason that zinc is essential for its proper working.

New medical tests have shown that immunological problems in children can be helped and corrected with zinc supplements. Read the section on zinc and if you feel you are not getting enough zinc, talk to your doctor about using a zinc supplement.

Secrets to Living Longer

People who live to be ninety or one hundred seem to share a common factor. They exercise in moderation—and, in fact, seem to do all things with sensibility and control.

People who live long lives don't overeat or undereat. They did not overwork, but they always worked hard and took pride in their work. They were not lazy. They seemed to have been very active, perhaps walking miles a day to work or in the fields.

Those who live long lives seem to have the same approach to the good and bad of life—they accepted their lot and trusted God to see them through. They learned not to fret. Casting one's cares upon the Lord is a biblical principle that also enhances a healthy lifestyle.

You're Only as Old as You Think You Are

One of the most important things you can do to successfully cope with aging (besides knowing God, eating right, and exercising regularly) is to know and like yourself. Accept who you are and realize that everything has its own beauty and value. Every woman possesses her own individual assets and worth.

Scripture tells us, "Godliness with contentment is great gain" (1 Timothy 6:6, NIV). Contentment is defined as an uncomplaining acceptance of one's life. To accept our lives and to live according to God's laws will reap great blessings in this life and in the life to come. If you have the beauty of the Lord Jesus Christ within you, your outward appearance will reflect it.

If you don't harness your thoughts; if you don't control the way you live, exercise, and eat; if you don't have a positive outlook about yourself and others, you will find old age upon you before it's even time. And it will be just as bad as you thought it would be.

Don't dare let anyone label you as old or even as elderly if you don't like to hear it and especially if hearing it makes you "feel" old. Age is merely a measure of time and has nothing to do with the mind and spirit of a person. If you believe you are old, you will act old, and you will look old. "For as he thinketh in his heart, so is he" (Proverbs 23:7, KJV).

27

Your Journey to Fitness

Today, at forty-seven years of age, I am in excellent shape and health. This came about through faith and commitment to a program of proper nutrition and regular exercise that I have been following for twenty years. I no longer suffer from any of the allergies or sicknesses that plagued me when I was in my twenties.

People often believe they must, through their own efforts, muster up enough self-control to harness their eating habits. They place faith, self-control, diet, and exercise in a row as their plan for losing weight and getting healthy.

Not me. First, God, through His Holy Spirit, made me sick to death over the weight I had gained. He made me see what was happening in my life as I reached for available food to cope with pressure. I realized that I knew how to exercise and eat right, and I knew that the power in me, through the Holy Spirit, was greater than anything in this world.

I acknowledged that the ball was back in my court. God expected me to put forth the effort that would burn calories, reshape my body and my eating habits, and restore my health and vigor. God showed me how to get my life back in proper order. This is the self-control that came about through the working of the Holy Spirit in my life. Remember, the Holy Spirit convicts us of sin, and through the intellect God has given us, we go forward as Christian soldiers effecting the work that must be done.

Are You Killing Yourself?

Are you like I was? Are you literally killing yourself because of your poor eating and living habits? Can you picture, with me, a new you? A fit, trim healthy person inside who is longing for a chance to emerge and develop? Your attitude and your faith will play key roles in your journey to health and fitness.

Ask yourself, "Are my health problems the result of my own abuses to my body through improper thought, diet, and exercise?" Be honest with yourself and God. When trouble comes, do you lean on the Lord, your brothers and sisters in Christ, food, drugs, or alcohol?

Your kitchen can become the devil's workshop! Is that where you go when something is troubling you? We need to get to the source of our problems and deal with them. In other words, deal with problems—don't eat them. We need to recognize stumbling blocks in our lives and see the areas where Satan is attacking us.

God designed us so that if we use wisdom and care, our bodies will run smoothly. A fit body comes from the inside out and is a direct result of determination. We must feel, "I am worth this. Exercising and eating right are not wasted time and effort. I am pleasing God and giving myself the gifts of health and fitness."

If we abuse our bodies with bad habits and improper nutrition, they will become sick. The first step to fitness and health is to determine what we are doing wrong and work intelligently to correct them with God's help. Seeking the advice and counsel of a health and fitness coach like myself is a very intelligent way to begin your journey to fitness.

Healthy Minds and Bodies

As the body is being made fit, our minds and spirits need strengthened, too. The body and mind are clearly linked. Grief, anxiety, unforgiveness, and guilt can lead to a breakdown of your health despite your best efforts to eat and exercise correctly. A tormented spirit, a soul without the peace of God, will never be able to maintain health and fitness for long. Many diseases are solely the result of mental depression and anguish.

Some people live in such a state of fear that the slightest exposure to illness affects their whole system. Then they end up becoming sick just as they feared. This happened to Job in the Old Testament, and he even confessed that the very thing he feared most had come upon him.

How much better off we would be if we had the courage and hope that comes from knowing Jesus Christ instead of the dread and fear of one without hope.

Laughter—The Best Medicine

The result of a healthy spirit is a healthy body. Even Scripture states "A merry heart doeth good like a medicine" (Proverbs 17:22, KJV).

How can we have a merry heart? By trusting in the Lord and by seeking to please Him in all we say and do. Scripture promises, "Thou wilt keep him in perfect peace, whose mind is stayed on thee" (Isaiah 26:3, KJV). Only in Christ do we find the hope, courage, and peace that is needed to have a truly healthy, fit body. True joy comes from the heart, not from another person or circumstance.

One of my viewers sent me a story I want to share with you. During an elegant party, a beautifully dressed woman went to the ladies' lounge and accidentally hooked the toilet paper with the heel of her shoe. As she returned to the ballroom, she glanced down and was aghast to see twenty feet of bathroom tissue trailing her. She was so embarrassed she could have died! But every time she told the story, she laughed long and hard, and the pain of that awful moment was relieved.

A hearty laugh is a form of internal jogging, a mini-workout that produces many of the same mood-elevating and tension-reducing effects of exercise. Laughing burns about two calories a minute.

When you anticipate a funny situation, your muscles tense. When you laugh, your muscles get a workout all over. With a belly laugh, both your heart rate and blood pressure soar because your lungs rapidly inhale and exhale air.

When you stop laughing, your pulse and blood pressure drop below normal levels and your muscles relax. If you have ever fallen out of a chair laughing, you know how relaxed you can be. Laughter is so relaxing it can even combat tension headaches caused by muscle contractions.

Laugh Your Way to Health

Doctors say laughter can heal physical ailments. Norman Cousins, a writer and former editor of the *Saturday Review*, showed that laughter is hazardous to illness. He was suffering from a degenerative spinal condition that many doctors said gave him a one in 500 chance of survival. Knowing his illness was caused by negative emotions such as tension and suppressed rage, he wondered if positive emotions such as love, faith, and laughter had any therapeutic value.

Cousins began watching Marx Brothers movies and old Candid Camera episodes. Soon he was laughing so much he was disturbing the other patients. Laughter was an anesthetic that helped him sleep. Within a few years, he recovered completely.

Laughter stimulates the brain. There is some evidence that laughter triggers the release of endorphins, the body's natural painkillers. Remember the runner's high? The endorphins may account for that overall good feeling you have when you laugh and may also explain how laughter can deaden the pain of serious illness. Many hospitals have opened humor rooms where patients can see funny movies.

Your fitness agenda should include healthy doses of laughter. Here are some ways to add laughter to your life:

1. Share your embarrassing moments with others. This relieves the tension and pain associated with the incident. Basically, you want to develop the ability to detach yourself from a situation, step back, and get a different perspective on it.

2. Seek out people you can laugh with. Laughing often creates a tremendous sense of closeness.

3. Open business meetings with laughter. This will reduce tension and promote relaxation. People think more clearly when they are relaxed, and the meeting will move along more smoothly.

Filling Up with Love

When people feel afraid, alone, or hopeless, they often overeat. We can become ill just from loneliness. This void cannot be filled by people no matter how much we love them. Only God can fill the empty places in our lives.

The Savior never forsakes us. When we love and serve God, angels are dispatched to aid us. The Comforter, the Holy Spirit that Jesus promised to send when He went away, is working in the lives of those who are open to the Lord.

If we are children of God, nothing touches us that He doesn't know about. We do not have to worry and fret when the great God of the universe wants to be our friend. Jesus reassures us, "You are my friends if you do what I command" (John 15:14, NIV).

In our weakness, the Lord will make us strong, and He will be glorified in our lives. When we believe He truly wants to help us with our battles, whatever they may be, then we can begin to yield to Him.

We are on our way to wholeness and fitness when we learn to trust His guidance in our eating, exercising, careers, and families. If His eye is on the sparrow, He most certainly cares about the details of our lives. Seek to please God in all that you do. Cultivate an attitude of gratitude as He works in you and through you.

No one can be healthy and happy when living only for self. Learn to focus on others. Channel the love of God that you've received to those in need. As you cheerfully serve others, you'll discover less anxiety and more happiness in your own life.

Set Your Angel Free

Let God help you. Let Him guide you and give you strength and courage to develop the gift that is in you. True rest and peace come when we stop being afraid and learn to trust the Lord. Too often fear paralyzes us. Learning to trust puts us into positive action. As we read God's Word and pray, we will grow stronger for the tasks at hand. We can truly do all things through Christ who strengthens us.

Here is a list of suggestions to help you on your way to a new, fit you.

1. Honestly examine your attitude about taking care of your body—while at the same time taking a long, hard look in the mirror—and ask God's help in changing it.

2. Begin to think of the disciplines you need as "gifts," not self-imposed torture. Your ability to stick with an exercise program or anything else depends on a positive approach.

3. Envision the new self you hope to create being born little by little every day. Each day is a new beginning, a "birth" day.

4. Use Scripture to keep your attitude positive. I've made it through many strenuous workouts by remembering God's promise, "Everything is possible for him who believes" (Mark 9:23, NIV).

Michelangelo felt there was an angel trapped and waiting inside every block of marble he carved. There's an "angel" trapped in each of us, too. All we have to do is set him free.

Resources

The following publications have served as valuable resources to me in the writing of this book and in my study of nutrition and exercise over the years.

1. *American Health Magazine*
2. *Shape Magazine*
3. *Health*
4. *Better Homes and Gardens*
5. *Reader's Digest*
6. *Anderson Independent Mail*
7. *The Medical Forum*
8. *The Greenville News/Piedmont*
9. *USA Today*
10. *Jane Brody's Good Food Book*
11. *Aviation Medical Bulletin*
12. *The Health Letter*
13. *Prevention Magazine*
14. *Tufts University Diet and Nutrition Letter*
15. *Mayo Clinic Health Letter*
16. *Harvard Medical School Health Letter*
17. *Controlling Fat For Life* by Robert Stark, M.D.
18. *The Percent Fat Calories Tables* by Robert Stark, M.D.

To obtain copies of Dr. Stark's books, send:
    $12.00 for *Controlling Fat for Life*
    $ 6.00 for *The Percent Fat Calorie Tables*
To:
    Dr. Robert E.T. Stark
    444 West Osborn Road, Suite 102
    Phoenix, Arizona 85013
    (602) 248-7852

Product List

The following items are available for purchase from Beverly Exercise.

Videos (VHS or Beta)

Total Body Workout. A one hour workout tape with exercises for your entire body. These ballet type, stretching exercises are designed to shape the body, improve posture, and increase flexibility.

Hip and Thigh Workout. A one hour workout tape with exercises for the hip and thigh area (inner and outer thigh and seat). These ballet type, uplifting exercises will firm and shape.

Audio Cassettes

Exercise Audio Cassette Tapes:
(Exact photo instructions included.)

Total Body Workout. An exercise program for the entire body. Floor exercises only, low impact. No aerobics.

Hip and Thigh Workout. Hip and thigh exercises only. Floor exercises, low impact. No aerobics.

Nutrition Teaching Tapes. Beverly speaks on diet and exercise. These tapes are designed to teach proper nutrition and the benefits of exercise.

Tape 1   Introduction to health
Tape 2   More on eating right
Tape 3   Health helpers
Tape 4   Selficide (eating disorders)
Tape 5   Food abuse and diet pills
Tape 6   Fighting fat
Tape 7   Where's the fat?

Tape 8   Lose the fat
Tape 9   Cholesterol
Tape 10   Fiber and Starch

Beverly's Personal Testimony. Beverly shares her personal testimony and the exciting story of her road to good health. Her ability to overcome serious health problems provides an inspirational and touching story. This tape also provides the story of her spiritual rebirth and the birth of her ministry. Available in audio or video.

T-Shirts

Beverly's T-Shirt. This quality, light blue T-shirt is inscribed with Matthew 19:2, "With God all things are possible." Sizes: S, M, L, and X-Large.

For further information or to order, write:

Beverly Exercise
P. O. Box 5434
Anderson, SC 29623

(803) 224-2498
(803) 225-5799